African Flying Doctor

NOTE ON THE AUTHOR

At age nineteen, having graduated from a New York high school where he was singled out for the 'Award for high merit, for scholarship and natural ability, combined with selflessness, modesty, and qualities most representative of the traditions of American youth', and having finished successfully a year of college at an Ivy League university, Jeff Baker decided that he wanted to work for a year in Africa. His reasons: 'Unfulfilled by what I felt to be a life of passive learning and immaterial ideals, I wanted to make my ideals real through action—to learn from rich experience, to do something constructive.' With his parents' consent and best wishes from the university, he made preparations to leave home for Basutoland, Southern Africa, to work with Dr. Carl van Aswegen's young and struggling flying doctor service among the primitive people of Basutoland's remote Maloti Mountains. On the eve of his departure, the challenging letter on the following page arrived from the doctor □ □ □

the Albert Schweitzer Clinic

under the auspices of

BASOMED

BASUTOLAND SOCIO-MEDICAL SERVICE, LTD.

(Registered in Basutoland)

Tel. Mazenod No. 10,
Masianokeng.
P.O. Box 169.
MASERU.

CvA 17th September, 1962

Dear Mr. Baker,

I confirm having today cabled you as follows:

'Please postpone final decision pending contents of letter posted today' - or to that effect.

However much I appreciate your willingness to come to our assistance, I want you to know -

a - that Basutoland is a newly emerging African State completely enclaved by the Republic of South Africa, with its own peculiar political problems therefore, and right at the moment suffering the pangs of birth into independence

b - that although most of the room for free and constructive thought is at present being liberally taken up by responsible Africans, there still remain the pinpricks of anti-Europeanism with its concomitant suggestions of 'insecurity'

c - that Basomed for the above reasons cannot by any means be regarded as a bastion of permanency for volunteers who even with the best motives in the world come to the assistance of (this part of) Africa

d - that our own efforts although possibly brave are really negligible compared to the gargantuan achievements of men like Schweitz and Dooley, that we have just started really that we are still only embryonic in our development, and that you therefore must not expect another Mayo Clinic on your arrival here

e - that however much I know that you are needed here you will be coming to Africa at your ow risk in that you will have to find your own way back should for any reason circumstances displease you

f - that Basutoland needs you nevertheless and that if in these circumstances you are still prepared to join us, you would be welcome.

Yours sincerely,

Carl van Aswegen

68

African Flying Doctor

A YOUNG MAN'S LIVING JOURNAL

Jeff Baker

W. H. ALLEN
LONDON 1968

PRINTED AND BOUND IN ENGLAND BY
HAZELL WATSON AND VINEY LTD
AYLESBURY FOR THE PUBLISHERS
W. H. ALLEN & CO., ESSEX ST., LONDON W.C.2.
491 00210 6

Illustrations

Everything in this book happened and is true. As it is not my wish to embarrass or invade the privacy of anyone, I have in some instances changed the names of persons and villages; I have in no way interfered with the facts.

The name of the country at the time the following took place was Basutoland. I have left it as Basutoland throughout, although today Basutoland has become Lesotho, an independent nation.

J.B.

October 19 —November 20, 1962

I just cannot express the thrill of seeing the coast of Africa appear, exactly as the sun came up. Then the smell of that air when we stepped from the plane at Dakar—it smothers one with fragrance, rich and balmy with a lush scent of flowers as in a greenhouse.

Later, continuing our flight to South Africa, we were delayed for twelve hours in Monrovia, Liberia, by engine difficulties and taken to a hotel nearby the airport. The weather was extremely humid and the sun, through the mist, was flaming—but once again the thick air felt wonderful, even though it didn't carry the perfume of Dakar.

A river separated the hotel grounds from bush; as I stood by the water there was the modern hotel behind, and in front, just across the river, was lush growth dotted with a few thatched huts. In comparison the hotel seemed coarse.

The hotel grounds were thickly covered with grass, grass scattered with numerous wild 'sensitive plants', plants whose small, delicate, compound leaves folded together suddenly, as with fright, at a touch. It was lovely and peaceful, especially at night with the thunderous crackling of a thousand crickets which could be seen hopping everywhere around and upon one's feet.

There were huge plants, quite ugly, with knobby trunks and great, rubbery leaves. The leaf veins are as thick as fingers—ugly, but very much alive.

Yesterday, upon arriving in Johannesburg, I was met at the airport by Kevin Harrison from the clinic in Basutoland. He's a friendly and intelligent-looking man of middle age who was born in England but has lived and worked for many years in the Republic of South Africa; this country has become his home. He has been working voluntarily at the clinic off and on as book-keeper and general administrative helper for only one month, so he couldn't tell me much about either the clinic operation or Basutoland.

He did speak to me immediately about South Africa, about the beauty of the land, but has said little of the racial situation, evidently avoiding the subject; occasionally his words indicate a great distress over the policies of his country, but at the same time he evidences a great love for his home and an unwillingness to hear it condemned by those who do not know it well. I'm only a naïve stranger, and am intent on maintaining a proper humility with, at the same time, a careful, open watchfulness. I am not here to condemn, but hopefully to work positively at helping Dr. van Aswegen build his medical service in Basutoland.

Mr. Harrison and I will drive to that country tomorrow. Along with other scanty bits of information about Basutoland, he gave me an impression of the extreme poverty there. He says that in flying over Basutoland one can see a borderline where the healthy fields of the Republic suddenly end and the desolate fields of Basutoland begin. The Basuto people let their cows and sheep roam freely and therefore the grass is eaten to the root, quite ruined. The country is poor, receiving a minimal sum of money each year from England and the Republic of South Africa; to live, the people are dependent upon their scanty crops and the small wages earned by the numerous men who go to dig gold, diamonds and coal in the Republic mines. The land of the Basutos is controlled by the Paramount Chief, His Highness Moshoeshoe II; there is no private ownership of land. The government is still British, independence not due for a few years.

Kevin Harrison told me, 'Thousands of the people depend on Dr van Aswegen.' As I began to visualize the doctor's work, he added, 'We'll be lucky if his service survives another month.' Startled, I asked, 'What do you mean?' 'It's a constant struggle,' he said. 'The work is overwhelming, the doctor's service is deeply in debt, and he has many enemies to his work. You'll see soon enough for yourself

This morning we began the eight-hour drive to the Basutoland border. The highways are excellently surfaced, and we drove with speed through the rather boring countryside of flat, dusty land which is the Orange Free State. As we approached the Basutoland border, the paved highway became a dirt road and the impressive blue Maloti Mountains, sharp and jagged, appeared in the distance. The mountains, where the doctor concentrates his work, looked more than impressive—almost unapproachable.

Soon we crossed the narrow bridge of one lane which is shared by the daily train and the few cars which enter and leave Maseru, the capital of Basutoland, and stopped before the roadblock which marks the border. The border post is that of the Basutoland government, the Republic having no border control though they are threatening to establish one soon. A smartly dressed Basuto policeman saluted us, exchanged a few friendly words with Mr. Harrison, and let us pass after we had signed a book.

We drove down the main street of Maseru, a parched little settlement with the rickety makeshift look of an Old West American mining townt,at the police station where I was to register.

In the centre of the town we passed a group of workers repairing the road. They were standing in a circle around a hole to be dug; one began a chanting song, and all the men joined him; at each downbeat—every five or six seconds—their glistening figures all moved in unison with one dig of the shovels. It's slow, but steady.

The street was lined with slowly moving women, carrying anything and everything on their heads: bundles, boxes, huge tubs filled to the brim with water—all easily and gracefully balanced. The women have a stately posture which pleases the eye.

At the police station I registered with little difficulty, the only delay being that everyone was fascinated by the American passport. We headed for the hotel pub to have a cold beer—our last cold beer for many a day, Mr. Harrison warned me. How wonderful we felt entering an unsegregated bar!

Later, feeling refreshed, we climbed back into the car and bumped eight miles from Maseru on a pitted dirt road towards the central clinic and Dr. van Aswegen's home. Mr. Harrison pointed to a small settlement beside the road—a cottage, two mud huts with thatch roofs, two prefabricated rondavels, and a small rectangular building of stone, this graced with a dry garden and some straggling trees—and said, 'Well, there's the main clinic.' I had expected to see a fair-sized hospital, despite the doctor's warning letter.

No doubt expecting my inevitable surprise, Mr. Harrison quickly explained once again that this clinic in the lowlands is not the most important site of the doctor's work; the doctor concentrates on providing a service for the people in the mountains who are not within reach of any other medical aid. The doctor lives here at Masianokeng, and runs a small clinic, but his primary work is in the Malotis where he has outstation clinics established through the villagers' volunteering their huts for use as examining rooms.

The clinic here at Masianokeng is small but well kept, a two-room building of dried mud bricks—one room for examining patients and the other for dispensing medicines. The doctor's cottage, and headquarters for his flying doctor service, is a beautiful building of three interconnected thatch-roofed rondavels of red brick; extensions, jutting out from the large round rooms, serve as bathroom, kitchen, dining-room, and small extra bedroom. Also on the clinic grounds are four smaller rondavels, two of dried mud, with thatch roofs and dung floors, and two prefabricated, of beaver-board. They house staff, patients, and stored medicinals. The doctor designed and helped to build his home, and obviously has taken great care with the grounds, planting beds of flowers and numerous, struggling saplings.

We were greeted excitedly at the car by Rosalia, a large, matronly woman whose dark and shining face radiated kindness. She has stayed beside the doctor for years, as his cook and general helper. She was very relieved to have Mr. Harrison home again, and was delighted by a simple gift he had brought her from Johannesburg. She welcomed me warmly and in broken English assured me that she would see that I was happy staying here. Her smile was all the assurance anyone could wish.

Mr. Harrison introduced me to young Josepha, a boy in his early teens, who beamed joyfully and wouldn't release my hand until we had shaken hands for at least a full minute. Afterwards he uncertainly offered his hand again to be shaken. When Mr. Harrison had taken me to the small bedroom off the doctor's room in the back of the house, and had left me for a moment to get settled in, Josepha came timidly into the room and we spent a few minutes talking. He speaks little English, and asked if I would help him learn; I promised that I would if he would teach me the local language, Sesotho. He was perfectly pleased with the idea.

He looked about fourteen years old, but when I asked him his age he said, 'Seventeen', adding vehemently, 'I am a man, not a boy'. I asked him whether he would be twenty-one next year, and, laughing, he said, 'I am a man, fifteen years!' Having felt me out to his satisfaction, he quickly made clear the purpose of his mission to my room by bumming from me two cigarettes. It was too late to resist.

Mr. Harrison later told me about Josepha: a month ago the boy's father died; Josepha came to the doctor and asked where he was to go and what he was to do. His mother, dressed in rags, later came to explain that her husband had before his death requested that Dr. van Aswegen should now be the boy's father. Josepha became the doctor's son, moving into the house; for help he offers around the house and at the clinic, Josepha receives money to send home to his mother. The boy is bright, has run away from school, refusing to return, and speaks very little English (though he probably understands more than it is to his advantage to admit); his belongings are a blanket, plus a few other pieces of clothing now, six cigarettes a day (he was able to mooch only four a day before my arrival), and an egg of 'silly putty' which he received from the American. A friend in New York had given me the putty before my leaving, and when I passed it on to Josepha he startled me by threatening to eat it like an egg.

As Mr. Harrison and I sat in the centre room drinking coffee later, Rosalia came in, and turning to him said suddenly, 'The doctor isn't in the mountains'. Her face cracked, and she said with a note of hysteria in her voice, 'I didn't want to upset you right away. The plane is wrecked, he left it in the mountains. He came here yesterday, he was all upset, and last night went to his parents.'

It seems that the doctor flew last week to a mountain clinic as usual, and spent the day seeing patients; during the night a violent storm descended and broke the plane away from its strong moorings, smashing it against a cliff five hundred yards away. In a state of acute distress, the doctor travelled three days on horseback to the lowlands, later going to his parents' farm in the Republic to calm himself.

Mr. Harrison explained to me that the aeroplane, which was recently donated to BASOMED by the Oxford Committee for

Famine Relief, and which the doctor—an excellent pilot—flies from clinic to clinic, is invaluable since it enables him to visit in fifty minutes, or less, mountain areas which used to take three to six days on horseback to reach. With the plane damaged, as now, hundreds of people in the mountains will be left without a doctor, and furthermore, if the plane is too badly damaged to be fixed where it lies or to be flown out, it will have to be disassembled and carried to the lowlands on donkey back.

Mr. Harrison, in a moment of discouragement brought on by Rosalia's news, tried to convey to me just what difficulties the doctor faces: the dangers of his constant flying in the mountains to short, pitted airstrips; the frustration and tragedy of patients expecting a doctor who must now wait for a wrecked aeroplane to be repaired; the hopeless feeling when a patient, almost cured, dies of infection after allowing a witch doctor to make cuts in her skin; the loneliness a man with the doctor's straightforward sincerity must suffer in troubled South Africa.

Dr. van Aswegen arrived yesterday from his parents' farm outside Bloemfontein, and we spent the evening talking over brandy and coffee. The doctor is a big man, strong and rugged, but with a gentle, almost pretty, face. He looked ageless. I found out long later that he is thirty-nine. From something tired yet distinctly inspired in the depth of his eyes one would guess that he is a man who carries the burden of a formal, thoughtful and profoundly serious mind. Though he is reluctant to talk about himself, and remarkably humble when forced to do so, he has an inspiring, respect-commanding force about him—indefinable but unmistakable and immediately sensed. His quiet power is almost eerie, and perhaps often vaguely feared by those in his presence.

He is an extremely ambitious man, steadied by a conservative BASOMED committee in Maseru, an administrative committee he established when he started his work six years ago in the hope that putting his work in the hands of local citizens would give it permanence. He realizes that this work must be done at someone's time and risk, and he has given himself completely; he doesn't feel that he has made a sacrifice in doing so.

When OXFAM donated the aeroplane, he learned to fly, and has since been using the Super Cub to reach remote mountain areas. The mountains really are almost inaccessible, even by air; the air currents are turbulent and unpredictable, and the airstrips are short and rough. The doctor has many times had opportunity to learn fully the hazards of flying a light plane in such territory. One day his engine stopped dead while he was flying over the foothills, and he only by luck found a rocky plateau on which to land. Numerous times, by improvising airstrips on cliff edges, he has landed in mountain villages never before visited. Now gale winds have torn his plane away from its sturdy moorings at the mountain clinic of Mafisa, smashing its tail on the rocks. Engineers are there today trying to put on a temporary tail in the hope that they at least may be able to tow it by air from the mountains. Meanwhile the doctor must charter private planes (when possible) even though it costs much more than BASOMED can afford. The operation is already deeply in debt—for how is it possible to be strictly businesslike about the costs of running a medical service when, most important, hundreds of sick patients are depending each day upon the doctor's help.

The doctor had things to tell me about the country: There are 'circumcision schools' near Masianokeng and throughout Basutoland where young boys—as an essential part of entering manhood—are circumcised. There have been some brutal cases; in many groups one of the boys, it appears the weakest, is sacrificed. The parents who step out of their hut one morning to find their son's or daughter's blanket lying by the door, signifying that their child has been the one chosen for sacrifice, accept the fact with sad resignation.

One day recently a boy of about thirteen staggered into the lowland clinic here at Masianokeng. He was suffering from severe stomach pains and an inability to swallow food. He stood shaking in anguish, but refused to remove his shorts for a complete examination. The doctor looked him over and could find nothing organically wrong with him from his partial exposure. Finally he insisted sternly that the boy strip.

He found the trembling youngster mutilated from circumcision, the wound badly infected. Questioned gently by the doctor, the boy hesitantly explained that to regain his strength against the pain and weakness caused by the infection, he had been forced to eat the foreskin of a friend; he had since found it impossible to swallow.

The local people also practise female circumcision, whatever that consists of. But the doctor explained that the initiation by circumcision is a vital part of the people's lives, bringing them much joy and strength.

Another recent case of brutality involves a nun from Quebec who had spent years trying to aid the people of Basutoland. One day in the middle of a township local villagers overturned and set fire to her car, killing and eating her, cooking her parts over her burning car in frying pans.

One day at this very clinic during a severe storm the patients insisted that they wanted a witch doctor to come and keep away the lightning. The people here are terrified of lightning; in fact, tonight during a brief but violent storm Rosalia was under the kitchen table. Among those who demanded the presence of a witch doctor was a trained, fully qualified staff-nurse. The doctor told them all to go ahead and get the medicine man if they liked. As the doctor explains with a blush, he, too, is inordinately frightened of lightning and is perhaps ready to try anything.

The witch doctor came speedily and surveyed the situation. He then reached into a bag he carried and painted large 'X's' all over the walls of the hut. The doctor's relief at seeing the sun come out was almost as great as his horror when its rays fell on the dark crosses. The 'paint' was a concoction made from human sacrifice.

The ugly, dark brown marks (which are still on these walls) caught the attentive eye of a passing policeman and brought on a harrowing hour of exhaustive questioning about their origin. Finally the policeman left, angrily and loudly wondering what sort of medicine the doctor practises and threatening severe punishment should he see such marks again.

Medicine murder, or *diretle*, from which a witch doctor gleans such medicines, not only still exists but is on the rise. The doctor recently was forced to testify in a case over a young herd-boy who was killed for medicine. The ugly process is to skin the body alive, and then to use the blood and organs as a remedy for the presence of evil, whether that evil be a plague on the health of the people or a famine on the land. The clothing (blanket) or some other possession of the dead is left on his family's doorstep, for their acceptance of his death.

These things are difficult or impossible to combat; the British government can do nothing significant to stop such practices—

though they insist on punishing primitive, perhaps innocent, customs with irrelevant Western law—and the people generally accept the situation. The doctor mentioned that it is inevitable that one day the boy here—Josepha—will just leave suddenly and we will know that he has gone off to a circumcision school. It's an important step in his life, crucial to his growth in Basuto society.

There is of course the good with the bad: the baby in a hut across the clinic grounds who was given up for dead by her mother and is now recovering from a vicious case of tuberculosis; the little herd-boys, only three and four years old, herding with pride many huge cows; the people who are being cured when ill by the doctor; the doctor's practical dream of bringing health and self-respect to these people through self-help; the happy, undefensive simplicity of many of the people here; the perceptive awareness of others.

And there is the warm smile of the ten-year-old girl at the clinic who, you note with a shock, has only sticks for legs because of polio, but who is smiling anyway.

The doctor decided it best that I should get an immediate taste of our work and of life in the mountains by going for a week or two to the clinic of Mafisa. He chose Mafisa because it is a relatively tame place with a large trading shop nearby, and also because he is considering shifting the location of the Mafisa clinic site and wants me to look around for possibilities and discuss the matter with the local people. He hopes soon to see the clinic run by the people of the community, their medical service eventually reaching a point of self-sufficiency; I am to speak to them about the importance of self-help.

Mr. Harrison drove me to the Maseru aerodrome this afternoon and a pilot and I took off for Mafisa in a one-engine Lockheed. Because of the presence of the trading shop, there is near the village a relatively long airstrip which can accommodate so large a plane. Before we even reached the escarpment of the mountains, however, we could see that it was impossible to circumvent the huge storm clouds approaching from the east. Just as the pilot turned the plane back towards Maseru, the edge of the storm reached us and we were completely blinded and deafened by the rain. We made it home, however, and tomorrow morning just after sunrise we will try again.

Never having flown in a light plane before, and having heard so much about the terrors of flying in the mountains, I found myself at first frightened, but after a few moments in the air it all seemed mild enough. Turning back was a disappointment.

Looking down from an aeroplane one is especially stricken with the desolation of this land: mile after mile of baked earth, cut by ragged teeth marks of erosion, scattered with clusters of mud-hut villages and parched fields. The mountains sit ominously in the distance, another world.

We awoke at five a.m. to find the weather cloudless, Mr. Harrison drove me to the aerodrome, and the plane trip into the mountains was smooth. I was hoarse by the time we reached Mafisa because the pilot, a South African Nationalist, insisted on discussing race politics with his new-found American victim over the roar of the aeroplane motor. I don't know why I allowed myself to get into such a futile yelling bout; such discussions are wasteful enough on quiet earth. It is incomprehensible to him that a black man can have the same intelligence as a white man. He kept saying over and over, in explanation of why he calls the black man stupid, 'You try to help them, you give all you have to them, and then they turn round and kill you. . . .' In response to my insistence that this must be little more than proof that his attitude and approach are wrong, that his giving must in fact be a form of taking, he gazed at me as if I were mad.

In this regard, a Catholic priest in Maseru told me an appropriate story the other day: a European walks up to an African who is relaxing in the sun by the side of a road and says to him scornfully, 'Here you are sitting lazily in the sun in mid-day. You should be working!' The African replies, 'Why should I work when I can relax in the sun?' 'So that you can make money,' answers the European, becoming impatient. 'And what can I do with money?' asks the African, humbly. 'What can you do with money! Why, with money you can get a better job, make more money and live more comfortably—and when you have enough money then you can find time to relax in the sun and enjoy life.'

I was met at the Mafisa airstrip by John West, a short man with a sharp face, his long pointed nose protruding over a bushy moustache. A trader from the Republic, he has settled here in the mountains; we drove to his house (on the grounds of which are also his shop and our clinic) in a small four-wheel-drive jeep. The plane flight was blissfully safe compared to this jeep ride over the rocky, sharply-curving mountain trail, the wheels riding inches from cliff edges. John concentrated on driving, saying nothing the whole trip.

We soon arrived safely at his place: a large comfortable house, clean mud rondavels for guests, a huge rectangular shop just bustling with people, a mill at which the people—for a high price—grind their mealies (maize), and a small brick building he has prepared for our use as a clinic. The actual village of Mafisa is about a mile from this settlement; the shop, however, is the area's centre of activity during the day.

At the house, both John and his wife Helen made me feel comfortable. As we all sat down for a cup of coffee, I jokingly explained, 'I'm sorry, I can hardly talk—I'm so hoarse. The pilot was an ardent Nationalist and insisted on arguing all the way here.' Helen West's pretty eyes widened with apprehension, just as John answered, 'I'm a Nationalist myself!' and went into a lecture about how it won't take me long to learn that there's no way to live with what he called 'these goddamned monkeys'. To my relief, Helen interrupted in a pleading tone, 'Now, please, John, don't start', and I quickly changed the subject.

I'm finding the language barrier a great problem here, but hope to quickly learn to speak Sesotho. The settlement is crowded all day with milling, mumbling people, many of whom wave to me and approach smiling to bombard me with rapid Sesotho—assuming I know their language and refusing to be persuaded of my limited knowledge. Many understand little of the existence of an outside world.

The language is hard not only because of its unfamiliar structure (it has a system of verbs, for example, which involves dependents and independents, negatives and positives) but also because of pronunciation difficulties. 'Q' is the click sound, and there are sound combinations such as lw, tj, qe, and tl; also, the vowels are pronounced differently from the English way, here flattened instead of rounded. It's a beautiful language, and even without that for an incentive, necessity and respect for the people whose country I'm visiting keep me working at it.

The people get a kick out of my embarrassed attempts to learn, and they laugh whenever I open my mouth to speak. It's fun though—they laugh with, not at, apparently not yet suffering the defensiveness of the 'civilized'.

The hardest thing to get used to is the peacefulness of this place. The mountains subdue thoughts of the rest of the world with their barren and strangely beautiful light brown and grey pitted surfaces. Everywhere in the settlement are the sounds of wild birds, wind, and murmuring voices—voices with the quality of muffled ringing—and there's a timelessness in the lives of the people. Horses, mules, sheep and chickens are everywhere, and only the chickens in their perpetual parody of people make any harsh noises.

This afternoon I went with the doctor's two medical dispensers, Mahapheloa and Tsosane, to visit the village proper, as the doctor had requested. We were greeted by the chief, distinguishable from the other villagers only by the relative luxuriousness of his blanket. In silence, he took us through the village. It is just a cluster of about fifty mud and stone huts, some of them with the walls caving in. None of the huts have windows, so the insides are pitch dark, and with few exceptions doors are made of thatch tied into sheets and placed over the hole which is the doorway. The people of the village must have been behind the thatch doors or in the fields, for the place looked quite deserted.

The chief turned us over to the village headman, who spoke a bit of English. He took us to a large cottage, square, and with small, ineffectual windows, and offered me a chair—the one piece of furniture in the room. I declined, not wishing to sit while the others stood, and, I'm afraid, caused a bit of embarrassment by my refusal. But the headman was quite friendly, and the four of us—he, the dispensers, and I—stood for fifteen minutes or so politely misunderstanding each other in broken English.

I felt dazed and lost, the surroundings being so very strange to me. As I wondered what was to happen next, for it was evident that we were following a procedure, I was led out to the veranda where, to my surprise, about fifty people had silently congregated, sitting on the floor and steps. I was handed a bowl of Basuto beer, a liquid, I learned later, made by fermenting corn meal. As I stood before their questioning eyes, staring nervously into the thick, chunky-textured fluid, the people around me began to laugh, at first tentatively, then heartily. With a burst of courage and with resignation to approaching dysentery, I lifted the bowl and timidly sipped. The brew was delicious, sour and starchy, and all the people roared with surprise and delight when I licked my lips and took a healthy second swallow.

A number of the villagers talked with me and we exchanged simple jokes, conveyed mostly by movements of our hands because of my inability to use their language. But a hush came over the crowd when the chief appeared. He came and sat down in the chair which someone had brought from inside the cottage; I sat beside him on the window ledge. The people clustered around us expectantly, and Mahapheloa, one of the dispensers, who is himself a native of this village, gave me a long introduction while the crowd scrutinized me with wide eyes as soon as they learned that I had come from a far away placed called 'America' and that I worked with Dr. van Aswegen. I was asked to make a speech with the headman as my interpreter.

I thanked the people for such a kind reception, and told them that I am here to learn from them and at the same time to help them do something for themselves, if they would wish it; I explained that BASOMED is very anxious to help them live in health, but cannot do so without their own co-operation and desire to help themselves. Self-help is unfortunately a new concept here, people being used to either charity or exploitation, so I elaborated on the importance of self-help with a view towards the future and a realization of the importance of self-respect in the individual.

When I finished, there was a long silence. I waited nervously. Finally the chief said thoughtfully, and ceremoniously, 'We are prepared to accept your help and all wish to offer you our thanks. You can see how badly we need your hospital at Mafisa. We will try our best to help you establish it.'

Questions were asked by the villagers: 'Do we have to work at building up the clinic and then pay for medicines too?' 'How do we know that after we've built the clinic you won't do what the missions and government do and say that people with no money can't use it?' 'Why don't you get the government to give you more money for us?' The questions all showed an upsetting lack of understanding of what I had been trying to convey. I again did my best to establish an understanding of the fact that there is more than a need for a socio-medical service here, but a need as well for self-respect and independence of charity. If the people build a clinic, they run it as they wish. If they want better medicines and better medical equipment, they form a committee to gather funds in the village for such. We will help where we can, if they indicate that they wish it, but the main responsibility is theirs. Furthermore, we are not a mission like other missions in the area, whatever those may be like, and they can trust us as much or as little as they please so long as they judge us by our actions, not by the actions of others. At that they applauded, and the question period was interrupted while many of them at once tried to step up to tell of Dr. van Aswegen's sincerity and good work as it has affected them and their families.

Additional questions followed the interruption, indicating that most of the people are impatient over the slowness of establishing their medical service. I explained that we are as frustrated as they with the difficulties of establishing and running mountain clinics, and can only try to battle ahead with them against obstacles of slow communications and rugged weather. Because it was apparent that they did not recognize the problems the doctor faces in reaching them, but rather blame him for bad weather and delays like aeroplane crashes, I tried to convey to them just how disturbed the doctor was over the delay in service brought on by his recent plane accident. They finally understood.

It was evident throughout the *pitso*, or meeting, that these people do not want to hear about BASOMED, the organization; they want to hear about Dr. van Aswegen, the first outsider they've ever felt able to trust.

One final question, thrown at me by an old woman, was something I had never anticipated having to answer: 'Where is it you are from?' she began. I told her, 'America'. She repeated her words, and to my repeated answer she asked, 'What is America then?' I told her, 'America is a country across the ocean, that way . . .' and soon had to add, 'An ocean is a river with the other side so far away that it would take many days to cross by boat; America is on the other side.' She shrugged me off as a hopeless mental case.

The question period over, the people all clapped their hands enthusiastically in unison, while singing a chant, and grinned at my confusion over the applause. The chief then turned to me and apologized that because of my sudden arrival not all the people of the village could be there to welcome and honour 'such a distinguished person'. I was stricken with awkwardness at this baseless praise, and told him as well as I could that the number of people present was far more than my due, but that I was glad so many people had come to hear what the doctor wished them to hear. The people laughed and began to disperse, many stopping to say '*kea leboha*'—which means 'thank you'.

Mahapheloa and I took another walk round the village, and this time people came forward to speak with us. We stopped to watch one man filling a large burlap sack with dried peas, a great bulk of them, and seeing my interest he laughed and asked if I would like to buy them. I assured him that so many peas would only give me indigestion. He was tickled by our mild exchange, and so was I, that people can be so unafraid and ready to laugh.

We parted with the chief on excellent terms, and the people—whether they had fully understood or not—seemed very pleased. I hope it gave them some incentive to help themselves; I certainly felt that already they'd given something valuable to me.

When I returned to the Wests' house I found John complaining bitterly. He had refused to see a chief who had dropped in from a distant village, and the chief as well as his numerous attendants were deeply insulted. John's belated apology, explaining to the chief that he had been eating lunch and hadn't felt like being disturbed at the time, did little to pacify the chief's anger at being snubbed and at the same time referred to as a 'bloody heathen'. Now John is worried about public opinion; a chief is a man who must be treated with respect.

All afternoon John shouted at me, his wife, and the walls: 'They're all a bunch of stupid monkeys, they have no brains at all, they smell rotten! I'll show them, I'll sit and watch them starve when the drought leaves them without food—and if they try to break into the shop I'll come out with my shotgun blazing, kill the bloody monkeys!' Towards the end of the day, John finally quieted, put his head on Helen's shoulder, and began to weep.

The people loudly call him '*Ntati Nku*', 'Father of the Nose', but below their teasing lies a deep bitterness, and with it, perhaps, some pity.

Dr. van Aswegen came today by charter plane, despite the cost of such flights, and ran a clinic. He examined fifty-five patients—a smaller number than usual because people hadn't expected him back so soon after his plane was damaged.

When the doctor first began this clinic at Mafisa a few months ago, he met with the village chiefs and their councils; they agreed that the patients should pay what they could afford for treatment. Before the clinic opened the doctor sent messengers to tell the people that no one would be left untreated because of inability to pay, but that those who could pay would be asked to do so. Instead of bringing in medical dispensers from outside, the doctor trained two young men from the local village so that, among other things, they would know each villager and his financial abilities. Amazingly, seventy per cent of the patients now give something for treatment; approximately forty per cent of those pay (with money, livestock, crops or labour) the full amount requested and thirty per cent pay part. If they cannot pay immediately, many try to pay for the cost of their treatment a month or so later. Of course there are those who come riding an expensive horse and wearing a rich man's blanket, saying that they are unable to pay—but they are not forced to pay; the handling of such problems is left to the community.

The doctor never touches the money; he prefers to let his clinic staff handle it. They are allowed to take money for their needs out of the total collected—but here at Mafisa they hardly take enough to live on, a decency of their own choice. Mahapheloa once worked for John at the shop and was fired for stealing; here at the clinic he doesn't even take what is his due. Dr. van Aswegen himself works completely voluntarily, having originally donated every cent he had into the establishment of BASOMED, and getting into personal debt.

The doctor wants to establish a new clinic, which would also serve as nucleus for an intensive social service, across the river where the airstrip would be only five minutes away; there is a good water supply and much more fertile soil, both for the hospital unit and for co-operative farming; at the new site the people could start fresh, with a pride in their self-established clinic and in themselves, instead of coming to a clinic built by someone else and given to them, a clinic centred at the home and business of a foreign trader. John is violently against any plan which places the clinic too far from his shop; and the nearest Catholic mission finds any intensification of the doctor's work repugnant. The mission priests are constantly calling the doctor a Communist for his ideals about co-operative advancement and insistence upon the (here radical) concept of self-help. The doctor dreams, and acts, towards a day when this clinic will be fully in the hands of the local people, with them hiring their own doctor and staff, as well as running the clinic and related social service on a basis similar to the co-operative concept.

At the clinic today, the doctor first visited a hut in the village where the nurse had placed a woman who was severely ill in the late stages of pregnancy. When we entered through the low doorway, we could just make out in the darkness a group of blanket-wrapped people sitting around a body stretched out on the dung floor. The patient's entire family was staying in the hut with her, helping to care for her; the people who ordinarily make this hut their home had voluntarily lent it to the sick woman, while they themselves temporarily moved in with relatives elsewhere in the village.

The patient was losing blood, and required immediate hospital treatment. After comforting the woman and instructing her family, the doctor went to his other patients; later in the day he had her flown to a government hospital. Before leaving the hut, the doctor promised the family that the girl would be well taken care of and would soon return to them, but outside he told me that, although he had no alternative but to send the girl away, because he lacked the means here for the necessary treatment, he often had cause to criticize the way in which his patients were treated when they left his care. Indeed, he had had the experience of checking about a patient he had sent to hospital from the mountains, only to be told that the patient could not be located; and not until he had spent hours demanding information did he finally hear, 'Oh, yes, she died three days ago.'

Today at Mafisa the patients filed into the clinic with pleurisy, tuberculosis (often in indescribably horrible forms), crippling malnutritional diseases, and such difficulties as inability to have children—a condition believed to be brought on by a magical curse.

One man with a broken leg arrived after having dragged himself for six hours through the mountains. A heart patient was carried to the clinic on a ladder become stretcher, supported at the ends by two of his fellow villagers; they had travelled for two days.

Numerous fatality cases whose families have given them up for dead are brought to the doctor to see if the death is by natural causes or by poisoning; when the doctor is able to cure many such patients in a week with 'wonder drugs', it builds the people's confidence in modern medicine.

There is, however, still a great faith in black magic. For example, the nurse at this clinic, Staff-Nurse Lebelo, suffers from a desperate vacillation between native and modern medicine despite her rigorous training. Last week, in removing a patient's bandages, she found a small lizard pressed against the healing wound. The witch doctors often place these harmless creatures, always underfoot in the mountains, beneath a patient's bandages to indicate the passing of illness from the body.

Nurse Lebelo carefully placed the lizard in a bottle at the time, and today brought it to the doctor. She held it up before him and exclaimed that the patient was now well, that the lizard had left the body.

The doctor gently chided her for believing that the lizard had crawled from the wound. He said, 'You know, Nurse, that it's not possible. You know that.' She almost burst out crying in her confusion. Shaking her head, she finally blurted, 'Oh, I don't know, Doctor . . . I just don't know.'

The doctor smiled, then teased her as he turned to me and said, 'You see, even my best nurse believes in black magic!' She burst out laughing in embarrassment—but on her way out she turned back to the doctor again and said despairingly, 'Really, Doctor, I just don't know.'

The people are gradually developing a faith in Western medicine, but at the same time they retain their deep belief in witch medicine (a belief which, incidentally, is often beneficial). Taking no chances, they usually try both.

Dr. van Aswegen works steadily all day, seeing patient after patient, without taking time to eat or rest. He sips tea constantly throughout the day, but never stops working. All this and more he does for no salary except that which provides the most basic necessities, and an occasional (here necessary) bottle of brandy.

He is troubled by this financial state only because he fears correctly that were anything to happen to him there would be left no payment policy to attract another doctor.

His manner with the patients is wonderful, perfect—a confidence well-founded in his manner, and a kind friendliness, with, as always, his almost formal seriousness. He's efficient, natural, warm, and gently firm—an excellent doctor and a fine man. If only he had some support other than that of his patients, who are dedicated to him as he is to them. It's painful to watch him working in a crumbling mud hut, applying medicines he would love to have replaced with those other doctors can today take for granted. But his work is still young.

One patient who arrived to see the doctor had travelled a full day and a half on horseback from Mpaki, where a government doctor visits once a week. I asked him his reason for riding such a long way while ill, when without any difficulty he could go to the British government doctor at his own village. Mahapheloa helped by translating.

The patient answered, 'I don't like the way they treat me there. Many people come here from Mpaki to see Dr. van Aswegen.' I asked Mahapheloa to clarify this, and he explained that though the government services are rich and well-equipped compared to ours, they are very impersonal; more crucial, the people, many of whom own nothing, don't get treated if they are unable to pay a high set price. The people resent this. They especially don't like the way the doctors examine them without asking any questions, and then don't say what is wrong and what the medicine they are to take consists of. Aside from the fact that these people, as people anywhere, resent impersonal medical service, there is in this society a special quirk: a patient will never tell the doctor what is wrong, where exactly the pain is, for he feels that if the doctor is worth his salt, he will be able to find the trouble. This is a test they put before the doctor for their evaluation of his abilities—certainly a precaution I would take if I were accustomed to consulting witch doctors.

When it came time for the doctor and me to leave, Mahapheloa and I went to my hut for a last talk and to relax with a smoke (after chasing away the Wests' huge German shepherd dog, who now follows us everywhere, and four baby chickens who had wandered in). We somehow found ourselves on the subject of marriage; Mahapheloa told me that he was just recently married, and had paid twenty-five cattle and ten sheep for his wife (that's an expensive wife here). Then he said that my girl at home, whose picture he had seen, was very pretty and asked if we had any children. I laughed and said that if I were married with children, I certainly would be in America now. He said solemnly, 'I thought perhaps you might be here because of being married and having children at home.'

We took a walk around the village so that I could say goodbye. People thanked me for coming and spoke with enthusiasm of the plans for a new clinic across the river.

They said goodbye with '*khautso*, *pola*', which means literally, 'peace, rain', or 'peace, and may it rain'. That's how tragically dry it is here; it has rained once, briefly, since April. When I arrived at Mafisa, John drove me from the airstrip across the river in his jeep; normally that river is so wide and powerful that it is a rough struggle to get a boat across. The fields are barren in the drought; this coming winter many people will starve to death, if they are able to survive until then.

When our charter plane landed us in Maseru, the doctor and I went to the hotel to see if we could find a lift to Masianokeng. There were four members of the BASOMED Central Committee in the lounge of the pub. We had a few drinks with them, one of them paying insistently; when anyone got up to leave, a drink was immediately thrust into his hands and he had to finish it before trying again unsuccessfully to be off. All were Basutos, the group varied—a doctor, a lawyer, a journalist and a businessman—and it couldn't have been a more stimulating evening. We discussed psychology, America, languages, and a variety of other topics, all the conversation sharp and witty. The doctor and I got home five hours later, tired but stimulated.

Before we went off to bed, the doctor pointed out to me that nearly all the committee members discussed everything and anything with relish, excepting the subject of our work. He added, 'It's the same way at committee meetings; perhaps they find the subject boring. They never come into the mountains to see what their organization is all about.'

I sketched a few fund-raising letters before going to sleep, telling of the doctor's work for people in the mountains, not concentrating at all on the organization. The enormity of his work amazes me; what would be just wild dreams for most men are in him, I'm convinced, a future reality. He gives his full concentration and labour to his ambitious plans, relegating obstacles —natural and human—to the petty level on which they properly belong. The extent of the mountain people's needs allows for no less sincere an approach.

There is a jackal living on the clinic grounds, and he's a pleasure to have around. He's completely wild and won't come near anyone but Dr. van Aswegen. One day last week he escaped, and immediately found himself before the bared teeth of a violent pack of local dogs who surrounded him, making all his superior ability at speed useless. Some herd-boys rescued him and returned him to us instead of eating him, knowing that we would pay them for the favour, and for two days the poor animal cowered deeper and deeper into an acquired neurosis, refusing even to eat his food while anyone—man or dog—remained in sight. When the doctor returned from the mountains, however, and said hello to the jackal, the animal came forward in an almost incredible display of trust and self-pity, burying his face in the doctor's cupped hands.

The doctor has an Alsatian, a beautiful and gentle puppy, who plays with the jackal. They never hurt one another, but occasionally get a nip at the other's tail. They chase about madly, the jackal at one moment running from the dog, then suddenly the dog running from the jackal, the chase reversed. When it finally rained a bit the other day, forming a puddle near the jackal's hutch, the dog—who had never before seen water outside his dish—was trying to eat the water as if it were a solid and puzzling over what was weighing down his soaked tail. Whenever the dog became too interested in the water, the jackal would sneak up behind him and nip his foot, starting the chase with both of them slipping wildly in the mud.

Josepha and I took the jackal for a walk on his chain yesterday. There are ant hills about three feet high, like earthen tumours, all over the land. The stuff with which the ants build them is so hard that one can stand on the hills. Josepha assures me that when the weather improves I will see such hills a good deal higher. Interesting, but a bit horrifying.

The rain we had was slight, but even so made the country look like a different place. I had been told that I was seeing the land at its least beautiful, but didn't believe it before this. After a bit of rain, hidden colours creep out all over the land.

Chief Mapetla, father of our Committee Chairman Joe Mapetla, and chief of Masianokeng, called in at the house today to visit the doctor. He's eighty-three years old, a well educated man, and a wise man; his conversation is rich with clever idiom and well thought out feelings of profound simplicity. For me it is a new and rare experience to hear deep thoughts about what we consider the small things in life, things which we take for granted and of which we're so unappreciative. He spoke for a long time about a sapling he had planted when the doctor opened his clinic here six years ago, and how it has grown and thrived through the seasons.

The chief was so old that I had to help him move about, out of his chair, down a step—he reached out for my support and leaned on me heavily. When I asked him how he was to get home, he rasped, 'I brought my horse'. I thought he was joking, but there was the horse, and somehow he got on it and cantered off as if he were a young man.

Yesterday while I was typing, Rosalia brought into my room a weird bug to show me. It looked like just a cylindical bundle of twigs, about an inch long, with a bush of woody fuzz at one end, the twigs converging at the other end. When she put it down the fuzz began to move and a black caterpillar-like head came cautiously out, looked around, and then began to pull its body forward. Rosalia laughed, as if to say that she had seen such things before but didn't really believe they existed (and still doesn't).

One reads of Dr. Schweitzer's refusing to kill even insects, and wonders whether he is living eccentrically or philosophically. I'm certain it's not eccentricity that drives him. Here in a primitive part of Africa it just seems common decency to step aside to avoid killing an ant, or to sacrifice reading by candlelight because the flame is killing one moth after another. Somehow all life of any sort seems to take on meaning; even the plants seem to throb intelligently. They belong here and have a right to live, an intense propriety—and every form of life seems as beautiful and therefore as important as another. When now I see crickets and lizards on the ground, I step aside—and, when occasionally I see a scorpion, I turn and run in the opposite direction.

My work here at Masianokeng is rolling along. Soon I will be in charge of almost all correspondence, necessarily doing the job from the mountain villages where I will be stationed. This part of the work helps me to learn the intricacies of the doctor's service, as well as putting me in a position of being personally involved in the formation of BASOMED policies.

Much of the correspondence consists of writing letters to hold off creditors. Business ethics mix badly with humanitarian requirements, and our financial situation is ominous. The finances can't be ignored, but there are too many more immediate and crucial concerns—like the patients.

Last night, a huge thunderstorm rumbling outside, the lightning coming frighteningly close, we were all feeling a bit ill at ease—especially the doctor, who cringes at the mere thought of lightning. After fortifying ourselves with brandy, and then feeling a good deal more relaxed about imminent death by firebolts, we entered into a conversation. As we refilled our glasses, the doctor asked whether we had heard his story of The Lion to Stalin. We sat back, and let him take our minds off the present.

In 1952, shortly after the doctor had graduated from medical school, he set up a small practice in the little town of Tennyson, in the Republic's Free State, a most conservative area. He had rented a small flat for his combination home and office. One night, as he was glancing through the classified section of the newspaper, his eye was trapped by an advertisement offering a lion cub. Feeling an irresistible desire to have a lion cub, now sure that it was just what he had always wanted, he answered the advertisement. A few days later two men showed up at his flat with the cub, and, overjoyed at the opportunity of ridding themselves of the beast, gave it to the doctor for nothing before he could protest. He promised faithfully to take good care of it.

The baby lion, whom he named Chaka after the famous Zulu king, moved into the little flat to live with him, his two parakeets, three goldfish, and a dog. He and Chaka got along famously, sharing their meals and later the same bed (in both cases the lion usually got the better half). As the lion grew up, however, and became a fully-maned beast, it became too big for the small room. The doctor was losing all his patients, and his friends began making excuses to avoid visiting him. Chaka had to go.

He drove the lion to his parents' farm outside Bloemfontein, and persuaded them to take care of it. They, as he had, soon grew to love the animal, and it took over the house. Their friends also began finding excuses not to visit, but the parents were willing to put up with loneliness. Even when the lion began to destroy everything in the house: chairs, rugs, curtains—everything—they remained calm; when Chaka chewed up the butt of Mr. van Aswegen's favourite shotgun, however, it took all of Mrs. van Aswegen's powers of persuasion to keep her husband from evicting the pet.

One day, while Mrs. van Aswegen was in town shopping, Mr. van Aswegen realized that he hadn't seen Chaka all day. He searched everywhere, and finally found the lion in his wife's bedroom where it had ripped apart and eaten all her possessions—homemade dresses, bedspread, bed. With a sly smile, he quietly closed the door to her room, went back to the living room, and waited smugly for his wife's return. When she did get back, and immediately asked, 'Where's Chaka?' he shrugged his shoulders and said he surely didn't know.

That night, at his flat in Tennyson, the doctor received an urgent call from his parents. When he arrived at the farm, his mother, shedding tears of anger, told him that if he didn't get rid of that lion immediately she herself would shoot it—if her husband didn't get to it first. Her son, immediately realizing the enormity of the problem of what to do with a fully grown, affectionate lion, muttered helplessly, 'But, Mother, what am I going to do with it?' She threw up her hands, saying, 'I don't care what you do with it! Send it to Stalin, do anything, but just get it out of here!'

The doctor sulkily left the room, picked up the telephone, and called the Russian Consulate. 'I wonder whether Stalin would like a lion for the Moscow Zoo?' he asked. They answered with enthusiasm, and soon things began to happen: special delivery letters and telegrams of appreciation arrived from the Consulate; long black limousines carrying fat, smiling diplomats of the

Russian government rolled into Tennyson and stopped before the doctor's office; a personal letter of warmth and appreciation arrived from Stalin himself—while the people of dusty little Tennyson stood with mouths agape. The Russian Consulate proceeded to have a large aluminium cage built, at a cost of £300, for transport of the lion, and prepared a feast at the consulate to celebrate the send-off of the doctor's 'patriotic gift' to the Moscow Zoo.

Amid popping of flashbulbs and crowds of people, the doctor proceeded with the animal to the Consulate; was filled with rich Russian food and hearty Russian vodka; led a large procession to the railway station where he put the lion onto the train and bade it farewell, getting his hand bitten in the process; received luxurious gifts from the Russian officials; and was put under detention for questioning by the South African government. They've kept a wary eye on him ever since.

The conversation turned to more serious matters before the evening was out. The doctor told me of a Roman Catholic priest who used to visit him at Masianokeng nearly every day—a close friend, and the Father largely responsible for the doctor's having nearly been converted to Roman Catholicism himself. Suddenly, for no apparent reason, the priest stopped visiting; he hasn't been around for a month. There's reason to believe that it might be because of pressure from the Catholic missions, which seem to be growing antagonistic toward the doctor's work.

At the mountain village of Machache, where the doctor has recently established a clinic, there is a priest at the nearby Catholic mission who, never having met the doctor, is openly accusing him of being a Communist. At Sehlabeng, a village about three days by horseback from Machache, a nearly disastrous incident occurred when the doctor visited it last weekend: on every airstrip there is a windsock tied to a pole; it is vitally necessary in landing a plane, for it indicates the direction and approximate intensity of the wind, always violent and capricious in the mountains. When the doctor flew into Sehlabeng on his chartered flight last Friday, the windsock was missing from the airstrip. The charter pilot wanted to immediately turn the plane back to Maseru, but the doctor insisted that they land; his trip had been put off so many times by bad weather conditions that now there were hundreds of patients waiting, many of whom had travelled days on foot or horseback to reach the clinic.

The pilot flew to a nearby village, where a column of smoke gave him an approximation of the wind conditions. When they flew back to Sehlabeng to land, one of our dispensers, Molefi Thinyane, was running along the strip below them with an unrolled length of toilet paper, trying desperately to show them the wind direction. Although he had been without rations for two weeks, he was also making signals that they should not attempt to land. His frantic efforts only made landing even more hazardous, but they were able to make a successful, if jolting, touchdown. The column of smoke, as it happened, was a sadly inaccurate indication of the wind conditions, for it was on a different level from the airstrip.

When the doctor and charter pilot stepped from the plane, Molefi explained that the head priest of the local Catholic mission had ordered the sock to be taken down the night before their scheduled arrival. Everyone in the district had known of the doctor's coming, for the week before he had dropped leaflets all over the valley. When Molefi saw a boy removing the windsock, he said, 'You can't take that down; the doctor has to land tomorrow,' and the boy answered, 'The priest told me to take it down, and not to listen to any objections.' In addition, the people of the village told the doctor that the priest warned his congregation that anyone going to the doctor's clinic will be excommunicated—that if people are sick they should go to the mission clinic (which is staffed only with an unqualified and unregistered 'nurse' and has no doctor).

Dr. van Aswegen's anger was matched only by his disbelief; he tried to calm himself before going to talk with the priest. The priest, whom the doctor had never met before, greeted him coldly. When the doctor asked him why he had taken down the windsock, the priest answered, without apology, 'I didn't know the plane was coming.' The doctor pointed out that every airstrip in the mountains is a vital emergency strip, for often forced landings are necessitated by freak wind conditions in mountainous country, and that it is madness, beyond being lawlessness, to remove windsocks. He questioned why, even if the priest had by some marvellous quirk not shared the people's knowledge of the aeroplane's coming, he had removed the sock. The priest answered, 'I myself had this airstrip built years ago, and I put up the windsock at the cost of the mission. It is not for the use of aeroplanes other than those bringing mission supplies, and as we were not expecting any supplies, I decided to have the sock removed.' He then went on to tell the doctor angrily that the mission had a clinic of its own which could take care of the people without help.

We have since learned that not only is the mission clinic operating without any qualified staff, but that they are charging high prices for 'medical service' and won't even see patients unless the patients can pay a set fee. Their primary treatment is the dispensing of that all-time mission favourite, 'medicated wine', a placebo of watered down red wine handed out indiscriminately to seriously ill people.

In addition the mission has a shop and grinding mill, for the services of which the people pay dearly. When a local man set up his own shop and mill about two hours ride from the mission—a fine, encouraging bit of self-initiative, so lacking here—the priest told his congregation that they would be excommunicated from the church if they went to the 'competitive' shop. Such threats are deeply frightening to a people who do not know better than to believe in the priest's power to send them to Hell fire.

We find the whole affair shattering, quite beyond the material effects of such practices. A man like the doctor tries to reduce the suffering of these people as much as possible, risking his life flying in the mountains, sacrificing his every comfort; and in addition to the discouragement of the insuperable amount of disease and suffering to be cured without proper funds or assistance, he must face the antagonism of men who are themselves supposedly trying to aid the people. This priest must feel we're a terrible threat to him to act in such a way.

I suppose we should try to gain the confidence of such a man, or at least to understand his fears. Quite apart from the personal issue, the Church is a large power in Basutoland, perhaps more influential even than the colonial government. The doctor's work certainly doesn't depend on their support, but it could be gravely endangered by their antagonism.

While the doctor was at Sehlabeng, a man showed up with an extra horse, and begged the doctor please to ride with him to his sick wife; he described her condition and it sounded serious. The doctor rode with him on treacherous trails to his home, and found his wife to be suffering from an extremely severe heart condition. At this altitude of 10,000 feet her situation was especially bad; she was all bloated and could not move. She is only about thirty years old. Now perhaps she can be helped; the doctor is going to try to have the necessary drugs dropped to her from an aeroplane. Molefi, the dispenser, will be riding eight hours to and from her home every other day—at the same time carrying on with his regular amount of dispensing work at the clinic. It's things such as this, says the doctor, not mission politics and petty antagonisms, that require our full attention.

I asked the doctor to let me go to Sehlabeng to help Molefi. He was reluctant, saying that this is one of the most primitive areas of the country, that I'd arrived only recently. But he promised to think about it.

Tonight at Masianokeng I went out to the clinic to see a little girl about three years old—maybe two—whose lungs are full of fluid. She was on the brink of death when her parents brought her in this morning, and the doctor and nurse have been doing everything possible for her. But, even now, she is covered with sweat and breathing with a horrid rattling sound. In the same dark hut are ten other people—sick people and their families. Outside, all around the clinic, are people sleeping on the grass and on benches, all wrapped in their one article of clothing, often their only possession: their blanket. The doctor is constantly upset that we can provide them with so little, and that we can only afford to feed them bread and milk. And to think that bread and milk is a real treat for them; most of them never have anything but *papa*—porridge made from maize.

When I went to the hut, the people joked with me; they're so accustomed to conditions we cannot bear to imagine.

Last week I mentioned a baby who was brought to the clinic struggling to live. The first night it had looked about to die at any moment, its breath just a death rattle. But day by day the child's condition improved. When I saw it on Friday morning the mother was ecstatic, for the baby was eating with good appetite, and on Friday evening she asked whether she might take the child home. The doctor had gone to the mountains; I told her to wait for his return and get his okay. On Sunday morning, the baby suddenly died. . . .

Later, the mother, who had quietly accepted her child's death with gentle sobs and a sad resignation, took the child's body home to her village for burial. When I went into the patients' hut in the evening, they were all quietly joking as if the baby had never been there. The past is gone, the future yet to come; they have the hard present with which to contend.

We learned today that the girl from Mafisa taken to a modern government hospital has not yet received any treatment and probably will not at all because the hospital has no blood The patient will probably die, and we're helpless against it despite all we wish could be done.

We received word today that our plane will be ready late this week. The doctor tells me that what I've seen is only a light preview of what is ahead.

He has definitely decided that he wants me to go to Sehlabeng. There I will set up a tent and hope that the wind doesn't take away my shelter as it did the doctor's on his last visit to that village. Molefi Thinyane, the dispenser at Sehlabeng whom I have yet to meet, has been carrying on alone and is desperate for help. It is a new clinic, set in one of the most primitive areas of the mountains. The main purposes of my trip are to talk with the priest at the Catholic mission about the windsock affair, and to try to establish livable relations with the mission; to get the people accustomed to our presence and attempt to make them understand the meaning and reasons for self-help; to explain what they must do for themselves if they hope to have a hospital and to search for a place to build a decent airstrip, as the present one is supposedly the worst in this whole country of treacherous airstrips. Also, we have learned that the air charter service in Maseru never dropped the drugs for the heart-diseased patient, and I am to bring them with me and see that the patient gets them regularly and without delay.

If Molefi and I find a new airstrip site, we are to ride for a day and a half on horseback to a trading station where there is a radio, or if the patient develops complications we must do the same—for we cannot use the mission radio. When the doctor's plane comes, we must build a fire by the airstrip so that he can tell wind direction by the smoke in the absence of a windsock.

The doctor tells me that there is not much he can say to prepare me for Sehlabeng since he doesn't know much about it himself, and besides, everyone handles raw situations as best he can in his own way. He seems almost apologetic about sending me to this place, a bit worried—which isn't very heartening. The one bit of definite advice he did give was that I must not ride anywhere alone; the trails in that area are the toughest around, and the people most primitive. Not speaking Sesotho well, I might run into situations which I couldn't talk my way out of. He said, teasing me about my anxiety to get out there, 'After a week there you'll be dying to do full-time administrative work at Masianokeng.'

As I've never before been on horseback, he gave me some advice for riding on the steep trails: 'Just hang onto the mane when going up mountainsides, and hang onto the tail when going down.'

November 21 —December 8, 1962

Getting into the mountains, especially to Sehlabeng, turned out to be a complex problem. When I arrived at the Maseru aerodrome on Saturday morning, and said that I wanted to charter a plane to Sehlabeng, one of the pilots who was standing nearby turned to me, saying for all of them, 'Are you crazy?' I told them, 'Perhaps,' and produced sufficient cash to persuade them to join me in my madness.

Saturday, Sunday, and Monday we found it impossible to land at, or even close to, Sehlabeng. It was hardly possible to take off from Maseru because of high winds. This morning, Tuesday, flight also looked impossible; none of the pilots would think of approaching Sehlabeng, but I persuaded one to take me to Semongkong, a village only a bit over a day by horse from Sehlabeng, and the site of a large, multi-directional airstrip. The owner of the charter service promised that as soon as Sehlabeng was clear I would be picked up at Semongkong and flown out. Perhaps later this afternoon, as the weather has finally cleared somewhat, or tomorrow. If no plane comes tomorrow I will see about getting a horse and guide; the problem with that, besides my having no riding experience, is that the rivers are so swollen from the rains that crossing them is nearly impossible. Also, it would probably mean riding through forty-mile-per-hour winds on muddy trails—a challenge for fools.

Presently I am living comfortably at the home of an old trader and his wife in the village of Semongkong. There is even a radio in the house. They seem kind people, and are certainly hospitable; they readily accepted my 'dropping in' on them.

This is a much more beautiful place than was Mafisa; Semongkong is a broad and, now that it has rained, lush valley surrounded by mountains coloured with rich greens instead of thirsty browns. Only a half hour's ride away is a waterfall, one of the highest in the world and a most beautiful sight. Weeks ago on the way to Mafisa we flew over the falls, but saw only a trickle of water; today when we dipped down into the valley to land we were right next to the falls which were swollen with thick brown rushing water falling hundreds of feet into a white fluff of spray.

I awoke this morning at seven o'clock, and just as I finished dressing heard the sound of a plane. I ran out to the airstrip to find Myers—the pilot who does all the flying into Sehlabeng. He asked, 'Are you ready to go?' I certainly was, and hopped into the plane, a Cessna. But when Myers tried to start the plane, nothing happened. Muttering and cursing, he got out and swung the prop around manually until finally the plane reluctantly sputtered to a start; he coaxed it to a roar, and with a sigh of relief started it rolling down the strip—in the middle of which we sank down a foot into the mud. With the straining of sixteen local people, who pushed up with all their strength on the wing struts, we finally found ourselves out of the mud and in the air, headed toward Sehlabeng.

I now know why no one likes to land at Sehlabeng. We flew into one of the most rugged parts of the mountain, the winds tossing the plane all over the place. When Myers banked the plane as if he were about to land, I couldn't for all my searching see an airstrip. We dipped around the side of a mountain, into a narrow valley, and there, across a deep gorge, was a towering cliff which was itself the beginning of the airstrip. It was clear that the danger stems from much more than the cross-winds which constantly blow across the mountain-top strip; the strip is short, so one must somehow touch down just at the very beginning, at the same time avoiding smashing into the cliff face. If, in avoiding the cliff, one overshoots the strip the slightest bit, he overruns the plateau and goes over another cliff, into another gorge. Myers, looking extremely tense, eased the plane in at just the right moment, touching down precisely as the land appeared under us; we bounced joltingly, but a moment later stopped safely at the other end of the plateau, quite in one piece. Myers fairly pushed the supplies and me from the plane, and took off again hurriedly as if not even taking a moment to rest the engine would give him added momentum for take-off.

I was greeted at the strip by a mob of local villagers, who gaped at me. Many men and women, and a sea of children, some of the children cute as can be and some of them grimy little things with dripping noses. The silence was deadly and uncomfortable, remaining so despite my awkward efforts at friendliness. However, a tall, strong-featured and bright-looking young man, Molefi Thinyane, came running over and greeted me warmly, pleased as could be to find himself with unexpected company.

He and I lifted our box of provisions from the strip, and the bottom fell out. A bag of sugar broke open on the ground, and after we had collected what we could, about twenty children formed a squirming pile and licked the grains of sugar from the dirt. We watched painfully for a moment, then went on with our work.

We set up the tent, a not uncomfortable six by eight footer complete with furnishings of folding chair, stretcher and sleeping bag, table, gas stove with no gas, and candles. It's fine except that the wind will probably carry it off any moment, as happened to the first tent here while the doctor was inside examining patients. Molefi tells me that it's amazing the way one can leave the tent at any time without fear of anything being stolen; our possessions might be blown away, but they won't be taken away.

We could get no horses because my visit was unexpected; tomorrow we will try to get two so that we can ride to the woman patient, and at the same time look for a place to build a better airstrip. There is a feast at a nearby village to begin a 'circumcision school' tomorrow, but we'll have to miss most of it. It would be a rare experience to see it—a celebration of the time when the boys of the area, young men of about eighteen years, go off into the distant mountains to be circumcised and learn the art of love. Before they go, there is a great feast with dancing and sports for which the people come from miles around. The sports involve everyone carrying two sticks and trying to hit everyone else. The idea is to be very alert and try to defend yourself with your own sticks when another armed person approaches you. As Molefi explained to me, 'It's a traditional game, and everyone loves to play it. No one tries to hurt anyone else, but some of the people are pretty rough.' I asked if some people didn't get hurt. He answered matter-of-factly, 'Oh, yes, tomorrow we will have many people with head injuries coming to see us.'

It would be wonderful if we could see part of the ceremony. People have been asking us if we will come, and the headman of the village, who is a close friend of Molefi's, has invited us to come as his guests. Molefi, who's from Bloemfontein in the Republic, has never seen such a ceremony first hand himself.

I met many people today and enjoyed them very much. Most were open, kind and frank; all say that they will visit us often and teach me Sesotho. I spent a couple of hours with the village headman, Morena Pita, Molefi helping to interpret, and we got along well. We discussed the difficulties we're having with the head priest at the local mission, and the chief said that none of the people like this priest—that all the children are afraid of him. He said that after hearing about this business of the windsock, he had sent a message to the priest saying that when he, the acting chief, had given the mission permission to use the airstrip he had meant that it was for everyone's use. If there is any more trouble he will forbid the mission to use the strip for their planes. Very upset, he proceeded to tell me that the priest has threatened the people coming to the clinic with excommunication—a word used loosely around here it seems—but the people have said they need a doctor and will go to Dr. van Aswegen anyway. The fact is that in their fear of coming to the doctor against the priest's wishes, they often delay coming until it's too late to save them. Molefi and I are going to have a talk with the priest soon.

Late in the afternoon, Molefi and I watched a man building a rondavel out of mud and stones for the doctor's work. He had a small sledge-hammer with which he was smashing huge rocks into smaller pieces for building. Most amazing to see him working with apparently limitless strength.

Two other men came over to join us, and the builder immediately started yelling at them. It seems that these men were supposed to be his helpers. Molefi and I settled the argument, however, and soon everyone was laughing: the rondavel is for BASOMED; Molefi had hired this man to build it, and then the man had hired his own two helpers. When the builder now turned to me and asked that I should make his men work harder, I explained that he himself had hired the others, and it is therefore his responsibility to see that they work as he wishes. He therefore resumed yelling at his men for not showing up until late in the day—a tirade which went on for nearly half an hour. Finally Molefi and I pointed out to the head builder that enough time had been lost without more useless arguing. All laughed and agreed, and the lot of us pitched into the work; at first they were astonished and disturbed that I was working with them, but as we went on they became accustomed to the idea and showed pleasure at it.

While we worked, a young man started chanting from where he stood on the top of a distant mountain, his arms raised to the skies. Women at the foot of the mountain, carrying large tins of water from the river on their heads, had stopped and were making high bird-like sounds in the direction of the chanting youth. Molefi explained to me that he is one of the boys to be circumcised, chanting of his bravery and strength, as is the custom; the women were ululating in praise of him. One of the men working on the rondavel said proudly, 'That is my son,' and realizing this, the head builder was more understanding of his not having come to work until late—for this a great occasion, the entrance of his son into manhood.

As Molefi and I, utterly exhausted by the unaccustomed heavy work, left the building site to go and have some food in the tent, one of the men said to Molefi, 'We are glad that the doctor has sent your brother to us.'

Upon our arrival back at the tent, we found a man waiting for us; he wanted us to renew the prescription the doctor had given him to cure his coughing. When I asked him how he was now feeling, he said he was fine—has been fine for weeks—that he wants more medicine to keep his cough from returning. I told him that if he gets sick again he should return—that the doctor gave him medicine to take until he got better, not to take for the rest of his life to keep the cough away. He laughed, went over to his horse, and presented us with a fat hen from his saddle bag.

Later, when we were in the tent eating a dinner of corn meal and canned beef, a friend of Molefi's—a fellow of about twenty named Majara—came to the flaps and timidly asked Molefi if he could speak with him. At our insistence, he awkwardly entered the tent and ate with us; I made the mistake of handing him a spoon, realizing only afterwards that it served but to embarrass him further because he is accustomed to eating with his fingers. We gradually got him to relax.

He explained that he is upset because his girl just told him that she doesn't love him any more. We went about rebuilding his ego, talking of his other girl friends, and soon he was beaming and talking enthusiastically. When the subject of tomorrow's circumcision ceremony came up, he turned to Molefi in great shock and exclaimed, 'You didn't tell him about that, did you?' I laughed and asked him why not. He said that it's just terrible for me to hear about such things. I answered that if it's such a respected and important custom of the people, it certainly can't be too bad a thing for us to talk about. He finally agreed, laughed, and ended up joking, 'Molefi and you had better be careful that you don't get circumcised yourselves if you go to the ceremony.' Little does he know . . .

After dinner we dug into our precious coffee supply, and Majara put eight teaspoons of sugar into his cup. As we were drinking, Majara said that he and his brother want to learn to read and write. I offered to teach them, and he became very excited (though I doubt whether he was as excited as I was). I said that he and his brother should come to the tent every other evening, and he promised they definitely would—and added, hesitantly, that he and other people in the village are afraid of me. I assured him that I am as afraid of them as they are of me, that I don't know their customs any better than they know mine; he was tickled with this realization and promised me that I would have many pupils of reading, writing and counting. He said, 'The people have had trouble for many years because they cannot count their sheep. If they have a certain number of sheep and a few die, they don't know how many are left.'

Now, as I type, it is late at night, and while I work by candle-light, the wind, blowing through the canvas of the tent, keeps putting out the flame. It's a bit frightening being alone here at night, in this totally strange environment, with the wind threatening to take away my shelter and a pack of hungry dogs outside.

Before going to sleep I must mention one more thing: Molefi today took me to a windowless, dark, musty-smelling hut of a family whose baby of about three months had almost died last week. Now it seems to be recovering. It wouldn't swallow its food, and when the mother forced it to, it kept being sick. I saw that its head was severely scarred with cuts and burns in a distinct pattern, and when I asked about them, Molefi explained, 'The mother took the child to a witch-doctor before bringing it to our clinic.' When she brought the child to the clinic, she was in tears over her confusion about whether or not to take it from the witch-doctor and bring it to the new doctor.

I was awakened this morning at five o'clock by the crow of a rooster five feet away from my ear, right outside the tent. I had been freezing all night, and had not found any extra blankets. I got out of the sleeping bag, and nearly died at the cold; when I put on my clothes, they were damp and clammy. Once outside, I found myself surrounded by clouds, slowly rolling masses of thick fog. Molefi appeared beside me and just as we entered the tent, rain began to pour down again, filtering through the canvas in a fine spray.

As we were boiling water for coffee, the headman of our village, whom we now call simply 'Chief', joined us and said he was afraid we could not ride in this weather because the trails were muddy and dangerous—hazardous for the horses as well as for us. Molefi had arranged that the patient's husband should come for us with horses, but now it looked doubtful that he would show up. We were concerned over the patient's remaining without medicines, but Chief promised us that even if it were raining tomorrow he would have his own horses brought from the fields despite the danger. He says, however, that he fears for us if we ride in such weather.

Chief is a short man, little over five feet, with a hunchback. Though he is totally uneducated, he has a rich sense of humour and special sensitivity; like almost everyone I've met here, he is totally undefensive and has a ready smile, but unlike most of the people he has a penetrating quality and a sparkle in his eye as he talks with us. He, Molefi and I spent the morning in the tent in the small hope that the patient's husband might bring horses despite the rain. At one point Chief said seriously that the witch-doctors could stop the rain if they so wished. I pressed the subject, not knocking his beliefs, but trying to prove to him that the work of witch-doctors may be clever, but certainly isn't magical. As we went on, I told him the story of the Connecticut Yankee and his prediction of the eclipse, and flipped a coin to show him the simplest laws of probability; at the end of our discussion, Chief understood me but still hadn't budged in his beliefs. When I mentioned to him the baby with the infected cuts on its head, he said, 'Such medicine is dangerous, but the cuts and burns will protect the child when it gets older.'

We enjoyed our talk, and both learned a good deal. He was surprised that I wasn't condemning all the work of the witch-doctors or looking down upon the beliefs of the people. He amused me, and made me think, with the statement: 'The missionaries come here and call us savages because some of the chiefs eat people, and then they tell us to drink the blood of their god.'

Later, when Molefi and Chief had left briefly, I was joined by a girl and boy, both of them about twelve years old (I'm not sure, for few people here know their own age) and as many tiny children as could fit into the tent—plus a few more. We talked as best we could, and they helped me with my Sesotho while I taught them how to add and subtract numbers up to ten without using their fingers. The smaller children just stared at me, grinning and giggling whenever I looked at them. This is the first time so many have come to visit; before now they have only peeked into the air holes of the tent, running away frightened upon my looking back at them.

In the afternoon Chief took Molefi and me as his guests to the circumcision ceremony. We had to walk about two hours up the valley to get there because the horses could not travel in the mud. It was a thrilling afternoon. The boys hadn't come yet, so we were there about two hours before the actual ceremony started.

The people were greatly startled, but clearly pleased, to find a 'white man' there, and everyone greeted me, shaking hands and talking excitedly. Molefi and I briefly met hundreds of people, and when they got used to us and realized that we were present to share in the spirit of the occasion, they began dragging us into huts to drink and celebrate with them. It was wonderful: we sat in hut after hut, joking with people, drinking corn beer, eating eggs, bread, meat, and corn porridge. The huts are dark and smell of fire; at first we would enter and have to sit for five minutes blindly until our eyes became used to the blackness. Soon the hut would fill with people, and we would pass around a jug of thick, sour corn beer as we talked. After a while we would move on to another hut. There was much joking and making friends. In the few rare silences that occurred, one of the women whispered gently, 'Angel passing through,' as is the custom.

I was asked many questions: for example, one woman, worriedly putting her hand to the pulse at the side of her neck, explained timidly that she feared her heart was in her throat; she had been fighting about it with her sceptical husband for weeks. I pointed out that it couldn't be in her throat, for if it were she would most certainly swallow it, returning it to its proper place anyhow. She swallowed hard, and, putting her hand to her breast to feel for a beat, smiled her acknowledgment of my wisdom. The people were just great, and many have said that they will definitely visit us often—that they had wanted to before but were afraid.

The highlight of the afternoon was the time we spent with the head witchdoctor, or *ngaka*, of the circumcision school. He approached us, a tall figure towering over the group of men who stood with him beside the ceremonial fire in the centre of the village. He wore a doctor's white lab coat, had rings in his ears and a stick through his nose, his hair was shaven off and he had a clump of feathers attached to the front of his head. His face, coated with a thick layer of grease, seemed in constant grotesque motion as it reflected the flickering light from the fire.

We shook hands silently. He stood solemnly looking me over for a tense few seconds, then said, 'You are welcome. I hope to soon come see the doctor with whom you work. I don't dare go to another witch-doctor when ill.' When I asked why, he explained arrogantly, 'I am the head witch-doctor of Basutoland. Another *ngaka* might want to kill me so that he can become the head witch-doctor.'

Abruptly then he turned away from me and began to lead a group of men in dance and song. He sang a chant about how for years the black men have learned from the white men, but now they have the opportunity to teach the white men while learning from them at the same time. He finished the chant with a mixture of Afrikaans, Sesotho, and English to symbolize the mixing of the races. His racism was intense.

Having finished the dance, he walked over to me again, holding his body erectly, and said proudly, 'My name is Tsehla, but you may call me by my English name, "Seven Days".' I asked him where he had got such a name. He explained, 'I was studying at a mission to become a Seventh Day Adventist. But on the seventh day God spoke to me. He told me that I would be better off becoming a witch-doctor.'

Stamping his foot, he demanded that beer be brought. It arrived in a heavy earthen jug, and it was passed around the circle of men. I drank deeply of the chunky brew, and passed it on in my turn. Tsehla said to me, 'I hope you don't mind using the same jug as the others, but that is the way we drink in Basutoland.'

I assured him that I enjoy the intimacy of our all drinking together this way, and he exclaimed to the men gathered around us, 'What kind of a white man is this?' While I cringed, he conferred secretly with the other men, and turned to me saying, 'In Basutoland we give everyone a name. We want you to be called "Brother of the Basotho" and for you to be called this wherever you are.'

He then asked if he could examine Molefi, saying he was a bit worried about the way he looks. Just the night before Molefi had had a severe headache, and the aspirin he had taken was useless against it; he had explained to me that there is a syrup the doctor gives him which helps it. Also, Molefi had at one point mentioned to me that as a baby he had had a disease which, though pronounced incurable, had disappeared without damage to him. Now, Tsehla examined him, feeling his head, listening to his heartbeat, and looking into the sides of his eyes. He told Molefi, confidently, 'You often get severe headaches on either side of your head, and pills do you no good. Also, when you were a baby you had a disease which was supposed to kill you.' He proceeded to tell Molefi a few things about his dreams which Molefi acknowledged were true. Now Molefi is all upset and confused about Tsehla's powers. The witch-doctor promised that he would visit us at our home next week, and bring a sheep as a present.

We walked around some more, being pumped full of beer and

battered with conversation. Many people told me that I seem to like the people and that they like me also and will visit me.

Suddenly all the women started making high ululating sounds as the boys for circumcision appeared at the top of a distant mountain. The boys, aged twelve to twenty, filed solemnly down the mountain towards us with a herd of cows swaying behind them and the fathers of the boys behind the cattle. The fathers danced and sang, bursting with pride for their sons, and the boys chanted poetry of their own bravery. The air throbbed with their din.

When they arrived, the boys were marched by the men into a fenced circle around the large fire. They began to sing in unison. They are to sing and chant all night, in preparation for leaving at sunrise to disappear into the mountains, there to perform secret rites and be circumcised by witch-doctors.

The fathers meanwhile stood in a circle of their own near the boys, and sang while slowly dancing and waving sticks in the air over their heads, clashing their sticks together at every beat. The women sat about the tiny village ululating their praise so that the air everywhere pulsed with the strange, exciting musical sounds. One woman, then another, jumped up screaming and waving knives about. Their high chanting and frenzied actions drove the men into more and more passionate spasms of motion as they danced frantically.

Chief, Molefi and I were standing by watching the ceremony. I tried to control my rising excitement. Suddenly I felt a tug at the leg of my pants. I looked down to see a woman of about fifty sitting at my feet, pulling at me insistently. I raised my eyebrows questioningly, and she said imperatively, 'Go! Go into the circle.'

I looked blankly at Molefi, then at her, then back at him. He was smiling rakishly. I pulled myself together and said, 'In my country we are circumcised when we are babies.' The woman answered, 'Then, if you are already a man, let me hear you chant your praises for yourself.' I told her weakly that I would rather chant praises for other people.

She looked at me with a blend of disgust and scepticism. She said emphatically, 'Then you are not yet circumcised. Go into the circle'

I stepped back as she exhorted me. Molefi went on grinning,

offering no help. She kept prattling at me, and I kept shaking my head. The argument might have gone on indefinitely had she not solved the problem by saying loudly, 'If you are really a man, come to my hut tonight and prove it to me.' I mumbled a vague promise, and looked at Molefi desperately. He dragged me away by the arm, laughing, 'In another minute she may ask me to come along with you tonight. Hurry!'

On the way home we met a few Xhosa women who were singing songs we knew, the same songs that Miriam Makeba has made world-famous. We were greeted by many people as we passed their huts along the path, and we were persuaded to go into a few huts for more beer. It's against custom to refuse what is so generously given—and because my stomach was so unaccustomed to the heaviness of the stuff, poor Molefi had to make up for my rudely small portions.

By the time we arrived home another storm was beginning. The lightning was everywhere. A woman called us into her hut for more beer. I had seen her standing near the tent numerous times, but before now she had disappeared every time I said hello. Her hut was pitch dark, for she had built her rondavel with the doorway facing the wind and therefore could not keep a candle lit inside. I promised that I would fix up a light for her, using a glass to shield the flame from the wind. As we left her, she very timidly asked whether I would visit her tomorrow. Later, Molefi told me that he had been told by some other women of the village that this woman is in love with me but is afraid to ask me to talk with her.

Now, night-time, I'm typing in the tent; there is a terrifying lightning storm forking down on the village, the rain is coming through the canvas in a fine spray, the temperature is below freezing, the wind is blowing the tent all over the place, and dogs continue to growl around outside despite the rain. While I type I'm drinking cups of chicory-coffee, made with only a half teaspoon to conserve our supply. I'm quite calm, only made nervous by those damned dogs and the lightning which keeps lighting up the whole inside of the tent right through the canvas. It doesn't matter really at all. I love this place.

I haven't had much time to write, and I'm extremely exhausted. We arose at five this morning and saw that it was slightly rainy.

We had decided, however, to ride to the patient despite the rain. We went on Chief's horses since the husband of the patient would not come until clear weather. The trails were thick with mud. My horse slipped a number of times, but didn't fall; the horse Molefi was riding slid on a bank, falling and landing on Molefi's leg, but he wasn't seriously hurt. We passed the Catholic mission and stopped for a moment to hear a group of people singing and see them dancing at a wedding ceremony. Then we rode on.

When a village needs medical help for someone, they put up a white flag for our attention as we pass. We stopped at two such places to see a woman with a lung infection and a child dying of starvation; at one point a man rode up to us with a child in his arms to tell us that it was coughing badly. There's so little we can do, for we have no radios with which to reach the doctor, the doctor at the moment has no aeroplane, and since this clinic is not at all established yet we have no nurse with us. We do our best, however, with our scanty knowledge, aspirin, and sometimes penicillin. We daren't do more. So we rode and rode, noted a plateau which looked like a possibility for an airstrip, and finally reached the village of the heart patient.

Upon entering her hut, we were immediately blinded by smoke from the dung fire they had burning inside; my eyes watered uncontrollably and I began to choke. Molefi showed me that by staying crouched near the ground one can avoid the thick smoke. Crouching, we could see the patient's family, sitting around the hut looking tired and discouraged; they brightened visibly when we told them that we had brought the medicines of the doctor. The patient was as the doctor had described her—a young woman, completely bloated but for her left arm and breast. She was lying on a blanket laid on the floor, a fire at her feet. We gave her the injection prescribed by the doctor, and told her family that they should massage her feet and hands to help her circulation, for she was icy cold. We can only do our best at this late date, and hope.

As we rode home we passed through the village where the wedding party was continuing, and were asked to join. While we were being stuffed with corn meal, beer and bread, we were approached by a man who spoke English quite well—the headmaster of a nearby school. He said that he had heard about me, and would very much appreciate it if I could possibly help out at the school—that there is a great deal I could do. I thanked him, and said that if the doctor decided I should stay at Sehlabeng for any length of time I would like very much to do such work.

Since it was getting late, we had to ride on. We should not have stopped, for now a storm came thundering towards us and began to shower us with lightning and icy rain. We were frightened of the lightning, not without reason, and rode like hell; I hadn't thought these horses could move so fast. The horses slipped constantly, but they balance better on the slippery mud when moving quickly; sometimes they just stiffen their forelegs and slide fifteen or twenty feet on the loose mud down the mountain-sides. Somehow we reached another village where the chief, after getting someone to take care of the horses, took us to his hut. The chief, an educated man, smiled at me where I sat shivering, and said, 'Do you miss having a motorcar now?' I told him truthfully, 'No.' Someone brought in two heavy coats and hats for us, and said he would send a boy to pick them up at Sehlabeng the next day. Seeing that such matter-of-fact kindness surprised me, the chief told me, 'Here we are all brothers.'

Slowly the worst of the storm passed into the distance, though the rain kept on. Refusing an invitation to stay overnight at the home of the chief, Molefi and I rode on towards home. The rain was uncomfortable and the trails treacherous, but, though it must sound contradictory, Molefi and I got a great pleasure out of this part of the ride. Warmed by the goodness with which we had been treated, we sang, joked—and just enjoyed struggling with the majestic nature of the mountains.

As we travelled, people came out of their huts to tell us which trails were safest in the rain; once two women called to us from fields about a mile away (sound travels clearly in the mountains) to tell us to turn round and take a different trail from the one we were on. Perhaps—judging from a later observation of the trail we were attempting—we owe our lives to their kindness.

When we reached the mission, at about five o'clock, we decided that we might as well take care of our visit to the priest, at the same time giving our poor horses a chance to rest. As we led our horses into the mission grounds, we were met by a young French Canadian Father of about twenty-five who greeted us with sincere and glowing warmth and then ushered us, at our request, to the office of the head priest.

We thanked him, and entered the office—where a strict and angry-looking man, a middle-aged French Canadian priest, glared at us through his wire-rimmed spectacles and said coldly, 'Yessss?' hissing the 's' like a snake. We greeted him and introduced ourselves, asking if we might please speak with him for a few minutes; he raised an eyebrow, and reluctantly motioned us to sit upon a wooden bench across the room. We sat in our wet clothes, shivering with the cold, and, explaining the condition of the heart patient whom we had just seen, asked whether we could possibly use his radio unit to send a mssage to the doctor. He went into a bitter speech about how his radio battery was wearing out, casting angry looks at the machine as if it were his personal enemy, and ended up not having directly answered our request.

We entered into a general conversation, Molefi and I doing our damnedest to be friendly despite his all too obvious suspicion; when the discussion seemed to have reached its easiest possible point, I gently brought up the matter of relations between the mission and the doctor, avoiding specifics of the windsock incident and driving towards the positive, concentrating on the vital need for co-operation. When I mentioned that certainly both the mission and the doctor wanted to provide the medical service that the people here so badly needed and desired, the Father spat at me, 'How am I to know whether or not the doctor is a Communist! You don't help a person until you know whether or not you can trust his intentions.' I was, fortunately, more shocked than angered. The chief's words of only hours before repeated themselves in my mind: 'Here we are all brothers.' I prodded the priest. 'If you can't have a bit of trust in people, you should at least not pre-judge them and deliberately hinder them in their efforts to bring medical help to a place where it's so badly needed.' I pointed out that I had good reason to be prejudiced against him before even opening his door, but that I had done my best to be open and friendly because I figured that a man who is sacrificing his comforts to work in these remote mountains must have some good qualities; I also noted that the local people help anyone in difficulty without ever questioning who he is—they trust that they should treat him as a brother because he is a human being.

The priest flew at me uncontrollably, yelling at me that the doctor had come into his office the day of the windsock being down, and had started talking business immediately without even having first a friendly chat. He said, 'The doctor is an extremely rude man—he acts like a Communist.' I answered quietly that the doctor is only human—sure he was upset, for he had just been nearly killed by the thoughtless negligence, or whatever it might be, of the windsock's having been removed; he had risked landing under such conditions only to avoid disappointing the hundreds of patients waiting for him, sick people who had travelled hours and days to reach medical help and were depending on him.

So we went on—finishing successfully in that we may at least have established a truce, even if we failed to open the way for co-operation. But how to co-operate, or even reason, with such a man? Above all, he seems to resent deeply the doctor's trespassing on his territory. At one point when things were at their worst, he said, 'This is *my* valley—the people need no one else.'

The horrible thing to think of is the effect such a man has over the local people; there are over 7,000 people in the area served by this one mission—people who have no other contact with 'civilization' except for the rumours they hear of Maseru and the Republic of South Africa from men who come back from the mines. He holds, literally, in this primitive area, the fear of God over them—and many believe every word and threat he utters.

After our return to the village, while I was trying to sleep, and having a hard time of it because of the howling storm, I heard outside a strange tapping sound. Everyone in the village was asleep, for it was about two in the morning, and I couldn't imagine what it was; it kept on, travelling around the tent—'tap, tap, tap,' a metallic noise. I was afraid to go out to look, for the dogs don't know me and might find me appetizing. However, as I couldn't just sit there trembling, I finally unzipped the flaps a few inches and stuck my head outside. There was an old man, an elder of the village, hammering down my tent stakes with a rock—in the pouring rain and freezing wind—because he feared that my tent might blow away.

Yesterday I was able to stay in the village. Molefi and some of the local people asked me to go to a party somewhere nearby, but I wanted to do some work. When they had left I sank blissfully into the privacy of the tent and began typing fund-raising letters. Soon, however, a few children came along and nervously poked their heads through the tent flaps; innocently I encouraged them not to be frightened of me, and before I could realize what was happening, a mess of kids had crowded into the tent to watch me and talk with me. All day I was so mobbed with visitors that I could hardly breathe, much less work. In the afternoon, I finally gave up trying to figure out a gentler way of asking them to leave than by using the only relevant Sesotho word I know: '*Tsamaiea*', 'Get away' In a tone which attempted to say, 'I'm happy to have you here, but there's a time to be alone', I said, '*Tsamaiea*'. They did.

I sat for a moment, limp with relief, and picked up my typewriter to write a letter home. As soon as I hit the keys, people began storming into the tent again. They had never seen anything like a typewriter before, and the tent was immediately full of fascinated, exclaiming onlookers; it was impossible to get anything done. We did have fun; I typed out the names of the schoolchildren, and they became all excited. Then, upon being heavily persuaded, I gave simple typing lessons to a few of my favourite kids.

Though I had enjoyed the day, and had provided some excitement for a number of people, I was somewhat disturbed that I hadn't been allowed to work in peace. When Molefi returned, the old man (the same one who had been hammering in the tent stakes during the night) approached him and said that he was worried that perhaps the children and some of the women of the village were keeping me from my work, or upsetting me. Molefi came to the tent and asked the mob to disperse—until finally only he, two of our better friends, and I were left in relative peace. The small group of us discussed the matter, and I explained to them that while I like having friends and visitors around—in fact depend on them—I do need some privacy. They agreed, but after they had left I was feeling a bit guilty and afraid that perhaps they had misunderstood me; we are used to such different things, and have such different ways of thinking from each other, that misunderstandings can too easily happen.

Early in the evening, when I was really feeling wretched about my intolerance, one of the women who had left in the afternoon came to the tent carrying a huge plate of porridge as a gift. I was so warmed by her gesture and thoughtful sensitivity that I managed to eat much too much of the heavy stuff—but I forced it down with pleasure to show my appreciation.

Today we again rode to see patients. As we travelled, people shouted to us from distant fields, greeting us and then asking whether I am a doctor. When we tell them that I'm not, they ask whether I'm a priest. When we answer that in the negative, they usually yell, 'Then you're a doctor. Come and examine us!'

People now know we're coming, and wait for us, making the work over-strenuous; every ten minutes or so a man on horseback will appear on a mountaintop about half a mile away, and call to us that we must come to this or that village. Numerous people come riding up to us with sick infants in their arms—and, while we can sometimes help, we feel terribly helpless in our lack of medical knowledge.

Wherever we go we are conferring with chiefs of villages about BASOMED's plans for a clinic and the necessity and reasons for self-help. The chiefs understand readily, for they are usually intelligent, often educated, leaders of the people; unfailingly they are excited about having a socio-medical service which will be the people's responsibility. Chief Tatolo, the area chief of Sehlabeng, is calling a community meeting to explain to the people that they must help themselves if they want health and self-respect.

On the way home today we met a man carrying a most beautiful animal; I don't know what it is called in English, perhaps a 'springbok', or 'gazelle', but in Sesotho it is called a *letsa*. This one is a baby—very soft, about a foot long and two feet tall, with long delicate legs, tiny hoofs, a large round black nose, a rabbit's high ears, and gigantic liquid brown eyes—one of the most beautiful and graceful animals we've ever seen. We were fascinated by it, and the man, who said that he was planning to make a meal of it, agreed to sell it to us for five shillings.

We stopped at the mission to buy a baby bottle for its feeding, but the store was closed for the day. However, an old woman who was there with her granddaughter said that she would get the key from the head priest and send the girl over later with the baby bottle so that the *letsa* wouldn't go hungry. After I had paid her for the bottle, and thanked her, we rode home. But, later when the girl showed up, she had no bottle, and was crying. She explained that the priest had objected to our buying a baby bottle for an animal, though there were plenty of bottles in the store; she was crying for fear the *letsa* would now die. Her mother has promised, however, that tomorrow she will tell the priest that there is a mother in the village who needs a bottle for her child, and then will bring it to us herself.

In the meantime we've been doing the best we can to feed the animal condensed milk, using a forefinger dipped in the milk as a nipple. If the plane shows up this week (one is expected for the young Father, who is returning to the lowlands) we will try to persuade the pilot to take the *letsa* to Masianokeng as we are afraid it might here be eaten by dogs or rats.

Back at the tent, exhausted and irritated by the hard day and hot sun, I blew up at a woman who is constantly pestering us for tea. One really has to watch one's temper here; it's important not only for reasons of public relations, but also because one must never forget to make the effort of decency to remain tolerant and sensitive to people's feelings. It's too easy, especially in this strange primitive place, to become irritated, and too difficult to be constantly perceptive of people's feelings when it's so great an effort to dig through strange customs to find the individual beneath.

Majara and his brother came again tonight for another lesson in counting and reading, and really went at it enthusiastically. It was thrilling—they brightened visibly with the realization of their potential knowledge. Rather than accept our invitation to dinner, they said they wanted to go home to work on the lesson.

Chief ate with us tonight. We decided to dig into our rapidly thinning canned food supply, and cooked eggs, fish and bread rolled together into balls. We had to ask the chief to stand outside while we fixed it because he doesn't like to see sardines packed tightly together in a tin—says it's unnatural, and won't eat them afterwards. He won't eat tinned spaghetti either unless we cut it up into small pieces before he sees it, because he's convinced it's worms, canned worms. He's a very sweet guy, always ready to joke, and though he's serious in his beliefs he doesn't mind being teased about them.

When we kidded him about the fish, he said he would show us something to change our attitudes. He said, 'Tomorrow morning at sunrise a famous *ngaka* is coming to castrate a horse which has been acting up. You should come with me, so that the *ngaka* can show you how it's done, with special herbs.' Teasing him, we expressed our thanks, but said that we would bring along some spray anesthetic and show the witch-doctor the proper, less cruel, way to do it. Chief grinned and said, 'Bring it if you like, and if you aren't pleased with the way the *ngaka* castrates the horse, then we'll have another ceremony at which you can castrate *me* with your spray'.

We were up and out at five this morning to see the castration ceremony. Chief met us and with mock condescension led us to the edge of the village where a group of men were gathered. The herbalist arrived, this time dressed in a colourful blanket like everyone else, and stood a little in front of the small group. The unsuspecting horse was led before him. The men surrounded the horse and bound its legs with ropes, then stepped back.

Complacently chewing on a mouthful of herbs, the *ngaka* smiled at my especially pale face, pulled out a long knife and wiped it on his blanket. Leaning to the horse, he spat on its genitals, dancing around the animal as he kept spitting juicily in order to wet them thoroughly. He then bared his arm and calmly sliced with the knife in a swift, continuous sweep as one might carve a grapefruit. The horse didn't seem to notice its loss. Then the doctor spat on the wound again, the bleeding immediately stopped, and the horse, untied, walked off in search of a sparse patch of grass.

We complimented the beaming *ngaka* and acknowledged the mastery of witch-doctors. We assured Chief that he had escaped suffering the horse's fate by our spray, and he laughed.

After returning humbled to our tent, we spent the rest of the morning mixing medicines in preparation for the approaching day of the doctor's arrival. We were able to work quite undisturbed, having few visitors since we had spread the word that we needed time to work. When we finished, we went to see how the rondavel we are having built is coming along. It really is amazing to watch the men build it, smashing stones, fitting them tightly into walls, and plastering with mud made by lugging water all the way up from the river. Gruelling as the work is, they seem never to get too exhausted.

The woman arrived from the mission with the baby bottle and we fed the hungry *letsa*. It spent most of the day sleeping, but whenever some sheep went by, it would stand up with its forefeet spread wide apart for balance. We're afraid that it might have been taken away from its mother too soon, for it seems pathetically weak. (A few days later our *letsa* died, and was eaten.)

In the afternoon, Tsehla, the witch-doctor from the circumcision school who claims he's the head *ngaka* of Basutoland, showed up. He examined me, telling me things while gazing into a bicycle's rear-view mirror he had got from somewhere. He diagnosed my ills by saying, 'You often dream that a bull is charging at you', and 'you are confused because sometimes you think you are a black man', and 'your blood is heavy . . . you have a rash in your eyeballs'. I told him that happily for me he's incorrect. I never had such dreams or obsessions. Undaunted, he tried a second examination of Molefi, and, unlike the first time he had examined him, was now all wrong. He shrugged and explained contemptuously, 'I can't examine educated people. They don't believe what I say'.

His wife, one of many, and two sons, of about nine and ten, walked around the village all afternoon with jingling bells, clanking bottle caps, and furs about their waists. Tsehla explained proudly, 'They are apprentice witch-doctors'. They have decided to stay at Sehlabeng for a while, and it is a big occasion for the local people to have them here—partly because Tsehla is very rich and gives them food. I like him.

Interesting to note that in the evening a woman slipped into our tent and whispered to us that we had had evil visitors during the day—that the witch-doctor is bad because he gives people wicked medicine and charges them a lot of money for it.

We rode again this morning to see the heart patient and gave her the prescribed injection, but it's impossible for us to know whether she is improving. But the one improvement apparent to anyone is the clear encouragement on her face now as contrasted with the utter hopelessness of last week.

When we arrived back, late in the afternoon, we found the head priest and the other Father from the mission waiting by the airstrip for the plane. The head priest avoided looking at us, but we went over and invited them into the tent for coffee. There, while old stoneface glared at us, we chatted pleasantly with the other Father—who was most friendly, except that he seemed somewhat terrorized by his superior.

When the aeroplane finally came it circled four times and flew away without landing, the wind being much too high. The pilot should definitely return tomorrow morning—and we are hoping he might have some mail for us; perhaps the people at the charter service have been thoughtful enough to tell Dr. van Aswegen that they will be stopping here with an empty plane.

The witch-doctor spent the day examining everyone in the village who could afford his services. He has many riches, which he showed us in the afternoon: he has Vaseline (a panacea) in great quantities and numerous goat horns filled with grease from human sacrifice. I didn't dare ask whose. Along with these medicines he has assorted trinkets, valuable herbs, and two huge cans filled with sheep fat.

In the evening he bought two sheep from a local villager, and a group of men slaughtered them for a feast. Tsehla said, generously, that the meat was for the people—that all he wants is the fat, to add to his medicines. So there was a feast tonight on the lungs, intestines, stomach and other internal organs of the sheep. Molefi has a weakness for liver, so we called Tsehla and asked if we could buy some; he answered that he would not sell it to us, but give it to us—whereupon he clapped his hands, gave an order to his wife, and soon presented us with a plate piled high with beautiful—oh, so beautiful liver. We fried it in fat, and with Chief had a rare supper, hoping the while that we were not exposing our insides to liver fluke. Later we joined the others around a fire in the middle of the village, and were stuffed with sheep's lung, intestine and trachea; Chief sat watching me with a sparkle in his eye, sharing my secret as I furtively tucked inedible bits of meat into my pockets instead of into my mouth.

After the feast a man brought a drum and started pounding it as the people began to sing. The witch-doctor's sons put on strings of beads and danced frantically. Gradually they danced themselves into a trance, shaking spasmodically from head to toe, going on and on, never tiring. The younger boy, however, did finally slow down—it was incredible to me that he hadn't collapsed long before—and his father angrily demanded an explanation. Gasping, the boy complained of a severe pain in his side.

Tsehla quickly took a long knife from his belt and waved it aloft. His wife held the boy firmly by his shoulders, while Tsehla made two long, shallow cuts across the boy's stomach. The youngster stood stoically, his face blank, gleaming with perspiration.

Slowly, ceremoniously, the witch-doctor rubbed Vaseline and grease from a horn into the bleeding wound. The boy's mother released him. Instantly he jumped forward and resumed dancing at an even more vigorous pace, no doubt to avoid any further 'medical treatment'.

Suddenly Tsehla called a halt to the proceedings. He took a sword from his magic trunk, rubbed grease on it, and waved it over his head in wide circles; slowly, then faster, he danced around the fire, lifting his knees high in the air like a prancing horse. The man next to me explained that this would keep it from raining the next day.

The *ngaka* finished, and the general dancing and singing resumed. Then the men made a wide circle. The *ngaka*'s buxom wife jumped forward and began dancing alone as the men around shouted encouragement. Her monstrous, not unattractive, rear end lunged, revolved and plunged in wild gyrations while the rest of her body remained perfectly rigid. It seemed that there were some animal moving about beneath her swishing skirts.

The amazing sight delighted everyone, bringing forth laughter and cheers. The chief kept exchanging happy, and slightly embarrassed, glances with me and laughing. Little does he know that the dances I am accustomed to at home make this exhibition look tame and civilized.

Now it's 1.25 a.m. and I must go to sleep. It's a remarkably clear night, and the stars not only really twinkle, but seem to be oscillating towards and away from us. The moon is a sliver of a semi-circle, a subtle and graceful shape. Chief tells me, 'Now it is a sliver, a scoop in the sky. Gradually it will fill, and then it will overflow and rain will pour down for many days'.

Early this morning a plane arrived to pick up the young Father from the mission, and Molefi and I were disappointed to find that the pilot had brought nothing for us. Molefi is most upset because his wife in the lowlands is due to have a baby this week, and we have received no news; the least the pilot could have done would have been to call the doctor to say that he was coming here. Perhaps the doctor has got his plane back and will drop mail and a note tomorrow or the next day; if not we will ride to Mantsonyane and ask permission to use the trader's radio. That means a full day's ride to Mantsonyane, a night there, and then a full day back.

At about 11.00 in the morning a mountain policeman rode into the village. We talked for almost two hours; he was fascinated at meeting an American—the first he's ever seen. He told me that he could see I wasn't an Afrikaaner or an Englishman, and couldn't imagine where I was from. He had thought of America, but ruled it out immediately because I 'speak such good English'. He had once read something about New York, and kept asking me questions, such as, 'Is it true that everyone has five cars?' He then said that not many people in the mountains know of America's existing, but that the educated people in the lowlands like America very much and feel that the American government 'is doing a lot for the black man'. When I nodded with grim reluctance, thinking uncomfortably of the race riots taking place all over my country, he said, 'Yes, in New York all men are equal—black men equal to white men in everything!' I disillusioned him, wishing it weren't necessary, and in trying to give him at least the brighter side of the picture, found that it didn't amount to much.

When I told him about BASOMED, and our efforts to establish socio-medical services on the basis of self-help, he got very excited, and began to tell me how for years things have been given to the people of this country by do-gooders and schemers, but the people had never been shown how to do anything for themselves. He complained that the Roman Catholic missions not only don't teach the people to help themselves, but compete with and stifle those Basutos who show some self-initiative.

He became thoughtful, and then said, 'You know, my name is *John* Mohale'. He went on: 'Though I'm a Christian, I don't feel right about having a Western name. "John".' I was listening, and he continued, 'You know, when I die, and find myself standing before the gate into Heaven, God's going to ask me my name. When I tell him, "John", He's going to think I'm lying! He'll say, "You tell me that you're a Mosotho, and then you tell me that you're named John. That isn't a Basuto name. You're lying to me—you'd better go to Hell and burn!" ' As he spoke, his voice had reached a pitch of fear; now he became angry and said, daringly, 'What right do these people have to come to my country and say "We're right, you're wrong". They frighten people, and take away their right to think for themselves and be themselves; they take away our customs and our pride, and give us Christian names and fear'.

Before he left me, the policeman saw in the tent a picture of my girl from New York, commented on her beauty, and asked whether we were married. I told him no. He said emphatically, 'She must come here and marry you! It isn't right that such a very pretty girl and such a handsome man shouldn't be together!' I certainly don't dispute her being pretty, but . . . my hair hasn't been cut in two months, I have a heavy beard, and the skin of my face is a dark reddish-brown from the sun and wind. I hardly would dare look into a mirror, even if I had one.

This afternoon Tsehla sent his wife to my tent. She entered, looking worried, confused, and sexually radiant as ever. She told me, 'Tsehla sent me so that you should give me medicine to make me have twins'. She was half amused at my stupefied expression—and half upset by Tsehla's command, as she wants no more children. I stood awkwardly, unable to find any words, sharing her discomfort.

From across the village came a scream, interrupting our strange confrontation. Gradually the outcries became clear. It was Tsehla yelling, 'Twins, twins we want! Twins!' We could hear him approaching the tent, a crowd clamouring behind him. Quickly his wife and I stepped outside to meet him. I stood helplessly, trying to look innocent.

Tsehla stopped a few feet away and confronted me, the people grouped close around him. He was loud and wild, but friendly enough as he insisted, 'I want twins!' He was impatient in his demands for the 'twin medicine', and finally challenged me, 'Do you have the medicine or don't you?'

I hesitated, then winked and said meaningfully, 'Tsehla, I have just the thing'.

The crowd shrieked and stomped at my retort. Tsehla, not so amused, suddenly grabbed and kissed his wife roughly; she giggled and screamed playfully. He glanced at me, then broke into a guffaw and dragged her off towards his hut.

Also this afternoon, much to our dismay, people started arriving at the village to see the doctor—having heard the plane which came for the priest in the morning. Many had walked all day, and we did our best to explain to them that I am not a doctor and that the doctor will be coming as soon as the plane is repaired.

Seven women arrived, with food parcels on their heads and babies on their backs, having walked, barefoot, over the mountains from a place seven hours away. Now they are sleeping on the floor of the leaky hut we use as a dispensary; the place is full of rats and spiders, but the women seem content there. I'm afraid we have nothing else to offer them. When they arrived they kept insisting that I should examine them, refusing to believe that I'm not a doctor—for I'm white-skinned, and don't wear the robes of a priest, so what else could I be but a doctor? Finally they let up on me, grudgingly, and after having some coffee with Molefi and me in the tent, retired to the dispensary hut. Soon one of the women came back to the tent, and offered us some delicious corn bread, which we accepted happily. But, as she was walking away, she suddenly whirled around and said with the fury possessed only by woman, 'You gladly take my bread, but you won't examine me!'

Long after nightfall, a horseman showed up from Khubetsoana, two days' ride away, with a note for Molefi from Molopo Moshoeshoe, another dispenser who is laying the groundwork for a new clinic. Molopo reported that his tent had blown away in the wind, and then the night before he was to move into a hut in the village the hut had been demolished by lightning. After that he moved into a different rondavel, but while he was away visiting a patient, his new home was hit by lightning and almost totally destroyed. Now he is building another home, and staying with village friends in the meantime. He signed his letter with, 'May God help us in our work, Molefi!'

Yesterday morning I was half asleep when I was awakened by the drone of an aeroplane; I just lay there at first, not believing my ears. Then Molefi came barging into the tent, yelling, 'It's the doctor, it's really the doctor!' I did a quick job of getting half washed and dressed, running out to the strip just as the plane landed—our Super Cub, all repaired. The doctor stepped out, took one look at me, and almost went into shock. I've hardly ever been happier to see a face than I was to see the doctor's. He was beaming. He told Molefi, 'You're the father of a boy!' and produced a bottle of brandy in congratulations. The child is named Carl Hercules Tsonane Thinyane, 'Carl' after the doctor.

The doctor told us that he had just stopped for a moment on his way to Mafisa to bring the news of Molefi's child and to make sure we were okay. We had coffee and talked of many things; I can't describe how fine it was to see him again and to receive the news of Molefi's son. Before leaving, the doctor told us elatedly that he is proud as can be of us and that we are doing more than perhaps we realize by holding the fort here, preparing the people for a future clinic.

I had a few moments alone with him before he flew off, and asked him how things were going elsewhere and in general. He shook his head, and said, 'Everywhere our work is growing and the people are doing more and more for themselves—but I lie awake at night wondering how long we'll have funds to continue, whether we'll ever get outside help. And the government not only refuses to offer us support, but seems bent on putting an end to our work'. I asked what I could do, and he put his hand on my shoulder, saying, 'Let's keep working with the people. That's why we're here, and when we forget that, we might as well leave.' I couldn't agree more.

Since Molefi had been really worried over his pregnant wife, we were now high-spirited all day. The change that's come over him now that he knows about the child is miraculous. At five in the afternoon, we hit the brandy bottle and made a special supper —a treat: beans, eggs and corned beef from a can, extravagantly mixed together to form a flavour different from that of our usual porridge and beans or porridge and canned beef.

This morning we got up at dawn and rode especially quickly on our rounds; the patients were much better. We arrived back at Sehlabeng early, and Molefi went to see some people while I stayed in the tent in the hope of getting some work done. I was irritated to find that it was so cold I couldn't type because of stiff fingers. Then, as I tried to make my frozen hands obey my instructions at the typewriter, a storm broke with all the usual fury, and I was besieged by a group of giggling, dripping fourteen-year-old girls. It was fun to talk with them for a bit, but I was exhausted and wanted to be alone. I couldn't send them out in the rain, but had to sit and be flirted with.

To add to the general build-up of raw irritation, a man dropped in and obsequiously begged me for a cigarette. I don't mind at all giving away cigarettes, but his damn begging was disgusting. The tragedy of the country was in his pitiful character, and I was in no mood to face it. I gave him a cigarette, and he, bowing, said, 'Thank you, Master'. I lost control and shouted, 'I'm not your master, damnit!' He looked at me wild-eyed, then fled. I turned to the frightened girls, and poured out some coffee for them, for we were all freezing. Then, forgetting them, I lay on my back on the cot and fought off creeping claustrophobia in the crowded tent; I lay there silently swearing at the flies—hating the damn flies which as always were buzzing and crawling everywhere. FLIES! Everywhere.

But the day ended with a tone of warmth and humanity. First I was visited by a man with whom I had been talking recently about the possibility of his lending us an empty hut he owns for the doctor's temporary use as an examining room. He had before insisted that we should pay rent, despite my protests that we have no funds and that the medical service is for him and his fellow villagers, not for us. Today he came to say that he had thought about it and would lend us the hut at no cost.

Just after he left, a group of women from a nearby village came, bringing some dried peas and scallions—great rarities here, as people usually grow nothing but maize. They refused to accept payment, but I insisted that they should. They wouldn't give in, for they had brought them as a gift in thanks for our work and for our having once recently invited them into the tent for tea.

Later, after Molefi had returned, we cooked dinner—delicious eating with the scallions. Chief was eating with us, and when we heard the old man walking by outside, we invited him to join us. He came into the tent, and seeing us wrapped in blankets for warmth, quickly left the hut, saying he would soon return. A little while later he came back and insisted that we come to his hut. There we found that he had built a fire of dried dung bricks and placed straw mats around the fire on the floor for us to sit upon. We were moved by his kindness, and sat around the fire warming our hands, talking, and drinking corn beer until late in the night.

In the intimacy of the fire's warm circle, Chief spoke about the mines of Johannesburg, where he had once spent a year working; his clearest memories about that year were of the bosses yelling at him as he worked, 'Come on, Kaffir, come on!' He asked me to please try to explain to him why the white men get all the money from the mines while the black men do all the work; he was also very upset over a statement a white man had made to him: 'The sense of you Basutos is as short as your hair' He asked me if this were correct. I told him that I certainly wouldn't say that the Basutos are sensible, but that I know they aren't any more full of nonsense than other men. I tried to explain the phenomenon of bigotry, and the need for decent people to try to put themselves completely above bigoted reasoning.

Chief also asked me about the world—what is America? I told him as well as I could of the size of the world and its many peoples with their different customs, explaining for him what an ocean is as I had for the people at Mafisa—describing it now as a river with the opposite side so far off that it cannot be seen. I'm sure that he didn't believe a word I said about the world and the ocean; the idea of the world is nearly incomprehensible to him. Words about people, however, he quickly absorbs.

Chief, glowing with excitement, said to me, 'We have to spend a lot of time talking now, learning the truth together!' He taught me more than almost any man could by showing me the depths of thought one can reach through perceiving things with sensitivity and open simplicity.

Before we went to bed, Molefi made a strange remark. He said that he's glad I'm here with him, that he isn't here on his own; before I joined him he had been afraid of staying in the village. He says that while everyone is extremely friendly and gentle, people at the same time have strange and dangerous beliefs in this primitive society. I remembered the doctor telling me that I shouldn't ride anywhere alone. . . . Now Molefi told me that he is frightened every time he is told that a certain chief of such and such a village wants to see him, for it could at any time be a trap to skin him alive and use him for medicine. The gentlest people, our best friends, would, in all innocence, murder us brutally, at the order of a chief or witch-doctor. Such things have happened here before.

I commented as flippantly as I could that not only would we make lousy medicine, but the way we've been eating, probably wouldn't even be nourishing. All Molefi said, though true, seems so remote and impossible; it doesn't really frighten me, but just makes me feel more intensely than ever the strangeness of this land of extremes—and of man's savage innocence.

Chief pushed his way through a group of women crowded around my tent today, and came in to find me typing. He began to imitate me, typing on an imaginary machine while looking off in another direction; occasionally, after striking an imaginary key, he would wave his hand elaborately through the air with a flourish, mocking the way I unconsciously finish my paragraphs. As he continued his pantomime, he said, 'When I learn to use the machine, I will go on working while I look in another direction and greet people, just to impress all the women'.

Talking with Chief about almost anything, it is impossible not to laugh at his—well, his constant conveyance of a humorous feeling. His eyes joke. Molefi and I have finally found something to tease him about, and now he has no peace. He is very proud of the fact that he never drinks or smokes, but recently we found out that he has a mistress (a married woman of about twenty whose husband is away in the mines). She's as cute as can be—a lovely 'vice' to have.

On the day appointed, the doctor arrived early in the morning. Despite the early hour, fifty people were already waiting for him near the clinic hut at sunrise, and when his plane finally came into sight, everyone clustered excitedly around the airstrip.

He went right to work, seeing patients all day without any break, and working into the night by candlelight. The doctor worked in the donated examining room—a windowless mud hut, thatch roof swarming with rats—while Molefi and I dispensed medicine in the small dispensary hut nearby. Every couple of hours I brought the doctor a thermos of tea; when I passed the people waiting outside, where they sat around on the grass, I felt among them that nervous hush known to doctors' waiting rooms everywhere.

When the day's work was finally over, at about ten in the night, we were too tired to eat anything but a bit of the cake the doctor had brought with him. We had a few shots of brandy, sitting around the tent too tired to make conversation, and went to sleep.

The next morning, the doctor rode to see the heart patient. He found her condition improved, and made arrangements for her to be carried to Sehlabeng from where he could later in the week fly her to a hospital in the lowlands. When he arrived back he immediately started examining patients again. When a man in need of constant medication was carried into the village from his home three hours away, we spoke with the chief who immediately arranged for him to be given a place to stay in the village.

The doctor saw one hundred and twenty patients—each one of whom he treated with personal, caring attention, each to him an important individual. Once, near the end of the second day, I asked the doctor if I could watch him work for a while, and received his ready consent. As he examined and spoke with the patients, I could see the exhaustion in his eyes—for he had been doing this work constantly, every day, without decent rest; but he took the same intense interest in each patient who came before him. At one point, between patients, he turned to me and said warmly, 'It makes one feel so humble, the way these people come here with such trust'.

The next morning the doctor was anxious to get back to Masianokeng because of difficulties there. We took off despite a fairly high cross wind on the Sehlabeng airstrip. Later he told me that as we roared down the airstrip he had seen a young boy to whom he had earlier promised sweets for a favour, but he had forgotten the promise. He said that he had an eerie feeling as we took off, for the sad face of the child had made him feel guilty and seemed a mysterious indication that this would be an unsafe flight.

When we were safely back at Masianokeng, relaxing over some drinks, the doctor laughed and told me that many people at Sehlabeng thought I was the doctor and were disappointed when he said, 'Well, let's have a look at you'. That's because I was carrying the needle; the people think the injection is all important. Also, there was a woman who kept pestering the doctor, refusing to accept his diagnosis. Finally she had said to him, 'Doctor, I'm either bewitched or pregnant'. When he remained confused by this remark, she told him that she had been this way ever since she had set eyes on me at Sehlabeng. The doctor told her that she must be bewitched, and I assured him that he was correct.

December 9, 1962 —January 12, 1963

Yesterday a boy of about seventeen showed up at Masianokeng with all his belongings, and said that he is going to stay with the doctor and work for his keep. The doctor asked him to tell me the story of how they had met. The boy, named Sechlobi, explained: one day, a few months before, near his home which is in the foothills of the mountains, he had been riding a horse which was not broken in well. Suddenly the horse was frightened by something and went wild, tossing him to the rocky ground. Feeling an intense pain in his knee, which had struck a rock, he managed to crawl home to his mother. When his mother undressed him, she found that there was blood pouring from his body where a sharp stone had torn him open; his intestines were actually falling out. He couldn't feel any pain in his stomach, but only felt cold all over and hurt where his knee had hit the rock. His mother had put a blanket over him, and said, 'You must wait here until we can find a doctor'.

By luck, Dr. van Aswegen happened to be in the area—though he didn't have his medical bag. He rode to the boy's home, but finding him in such terrible condition, was nearly lost without his doctor's equipment. Nevertheless, he called together all the grandmothers of the village, collected what makeshift equipment he could, and using woollen yarn in place of nylon thread, a large needle for sewing leather instead of a surgical needle, and kerosene for methylated spirits, he sewed up the youth's gaping wound. Despite all his efforts he felt sure at the time that the boy could not survive.

Two weeks later, while the doctor was doing a clinic at Masianokeng, Sechlobi showed up, having walked fourteen miles from his mountain home; he complained to the doctor, 'My stitches are falling out'. Amazed by this miracle, the doctor removed the infected, rotting woollen stitches and did a proper job on the wound. The boy was fine.

After that, the boy often came to visit the doctor. He would sometimes come while the doctor was at work, sit beside him on the floor for an hour or two without uttering a word, and then walk the fourteen miles to his home, barefoot. Now the boy's parents have sent him to the doctor, saying that Rosalia should be his mother and the doctor his father. He will live here with Josepha, and go to school—where he hopes to start training to become a doctor. When I asked him why he had visited so often when it involved walking so far, and now had come to stay, he answered that in the doctor he had found '*ho rata*', love, and that he wants to stand by him.

Today the doctor told me of a new problem of large proportions. When he first started working in the mountains, before he had the aeroplane, he established a clinic at the village of Machache and visited it by jeep track. At first he worked at the property of the local trader, who, typically, wanted to have the medical service near his shop since it brings business. He had to leave finally because the trader was such an unbearable bigot. He moved the clinic into the home of the minister, Reverend Mohale, at the Protestant mission nearby—where it remained.

The doctor now fears that we might have to leave Machache entirely, because of the antagonism of a local Roman Catholic mission, despite the fact that there is much money and time invested in our clinic, the people very much want a doctor's services, and, though the place is reachable by jeep track, it is still very remote and has no medical service anywhere nearby. He explained that the clinic stands on a peninsula of land, surrounded by a river. On the same piece of land with the clinic and the Protestant mission is the local village, across the river on one side is the trading shop, and across the river on the other side of the peninsula is the Roman Catholic mission. The Protestant mission is sympathetic to our work, but the Catholic mission is so anti-us that we need a team of politicians to combat their trouble making;

the trader is also very much against our work because of the early dispute with him.

The important problem is the Catholic mission's waging a campaign against BASOMED, the same old business of threatening people with excommunication if they go to the doctor. Though there are plenty of patients to see him when he goes to do a clinic, Dr. van Aswegen finds that many others are afraid to come to him, and some of those who do come are, by the time they overcome their fright of the Church and see him, terminal cases.

In the hope of ending the antagonism, Dr. van Aswegen took time on his last visit to leave his patients and go see the head priest of the Machache mission. The priest told him that there is no need for a doctor in the area because the mission has a forty-bed hospital. When the doctor saw the 'hospital' he found it to be two small rooms each jammed with twenty cots; there was no doctor, but an unqualified, unregistered nurse in charge. The medicines this 'nurse' was using included streptomycin, tincture of digitalis, and morphia. Noting there a patient on the verge of dying, the doctor asked the nurse what was the cause. She told him it was tuberculosis. Shocked, the doctor asked what, then, if he had tuberculosis, was he doing in the same room with three small children? Upon examining the patient, the doctor found him to be dying of lung cancer.

The doctor told the priest what he had found, and suggested cordially that he would be willing to provide the services of a doctor once a week at the mission 'hospital' and would provide a fully qualified Staff-Nurse/Midwife to aid the 'nurse' now in charge. The answer was negative, co-operation impossible. The priest repeated, 'The people don't need a doctor here in addition to what our hospital gives them'.

We received a letter today from the Native Recruiting Corporation indicating that the Chamber of Mines of South Africa will probably donate money to us from their deferred payment fund so that we can buy two-way radio equipment, thus connecting at all times the mountain clinics with each other, with lowland headquarters, and with the aeroplane. Finally a bit of material encouragement! Radio communications would not only make the doctor's flying much safer, by enabling him to know weather conditions at all clinics and to be in touch with us should there be any trouble with the plane, but would also be of tremendous benefit to patients at each clinic who could, through the nurse, consult with or call the doctor in emergencies. We applied to the Chamber of Mines for this grant because we feel that they are obligated to help us—firstly, because our work directly involves the welfare of the thousands of men who go from Basutoland to the mines, and secondly, because the money they give out is payment deferred from the workers' salaries for the benefit of the workers.

The other major occurrence of the day is unpleasant and shocking: the doctor had a patient some time ago who was suffering from an advanced cancer; he sent her to a British government hospital, in the hope that they would attempt an operation. Today the patient came to us in great pain to say that the hospital had sent her away, finding her incurable.

I asked Dr. van Aswegen about this, and he told me that he used to send such patients to the hospital in Bloemfontein, where facilities were better—but to do so it was necessary to first take the patient over the Basutoland border to his parents' farm, then to coach the patient, who must be a citizen of the Republic to get into the hospital, to say that he worked on the farm. When one day such a patient told the hospital authorities, 'Dr. van Aswegen told me to say that I work on his parents' farm', it put an end to this life-saving scheme.

Lately I've had a lot of opportunity to spend time alone with the doctor. Often his discussions sail off into the abstract, but usually we are busy hashing out practical problems of the work. He seems to have accepted me as a right-hand man, trusting my judgement and respecting my opinion; the better I get to know him—and he is a difficult man to understand at all—the more I respect and appreciate him. His dedication and humility act as an inspiring guide to me in my work for him and in my personal growth.

Although it's nearly Christmas time, it's impossible for the doctor to take even a short holiday. There's just too much to do, our mountain programme progressing at a frantic pace. He needs a rest desperately; his flying and clinical programme alone would be enough to kill most men, but he has in addition to cope with the running of BASOMED and the antagonisms, the discouraging antagonisms, of those who are supposed to be sharing a humane responsibility.

This afternoon we were visited at Masianokeng by a Mr. Mohau, a school teacher from Machache who teaches at the Protestant mission where we have our clinic. For a long time we discussed the problems being created there by the local Catholic mission. He told me that difficulties have become even more serious: not only is the priest threatening the people into not seeing the doctor and nurse we have stationed there, but now he has aided mission representatives in passing a false petition among the people. The mission petition says that Dr. van Aswegen isn't wanted at Machache, and it has been passed round to illiterate people who think it is a petition to preserve the chieftain system.

By the time he finished telling us these things, I was steaming. Mr. Mohau, a sensitive young man of about twenty-five, is also furious; he tells us that the people desperately need Dr. van Aswegen, and want him to stay and help them build a hospital. They are very upset over the petition, so upset that they have gone so far as to send a representative to the government in the lowlands to investigate the situation. Mr. Mohau was sent specifically to speak with us. When I asked what he thinks is the cause of the Catholic mission's being so against the doctor's helping people, Mr. Mohau told me it's his impression that the Catholics don't want the Basutos to do anything for themselves or to have any self-respect, because that would decrease missionary power; he added that the mission hospital, which is useless medically, is apparently there in the interests of making money and converting people, not to cure people. If any others come to do anything for the local people, the mission considers them competition and resents them—calls them Communists and competes with them, threatening naïve villagers and exerting all kinds of pressures on the village chiefs. He concluded, 'The view of the Catholic missions seems to be that they must keep the people poor and ignorant, for once people have a better life and an ability to think for themselves, they will overrun the white people and become Communists'.

We don't know why we face so much antagonism; we know that various individual priests seem to have a distinct, seemingly personal, fear of our presence—but there are many subtleties in the total picture. I repeat Mr. Mohau's words and feelings because they are of special interest, representing presumably the viewpoint of the country's more educated people.

But, whatever happens, the people of Machache must have a doctor, and must not be denied for any reason the opportunity to advance in their own way. I have to go to Machache tomorrow with Mr. Mohau to find out what's going on; I'll stay there until around December 23rd or 24th when the doctor will pick me up in the aeroplane. Hell of a way to spend Christmas.

Headed for Machache, I'm presently at the lowland town of Leribe, after having travelled six hours from Maseru by bus. I'm in a hotel room, lousy but comfortable. Tomorrow I go by jeep to Machache, a trip which is reputed to be a horrifying experience, mile after mile of precarious jeep track through the mountains. I'll be meeting Mr. Mohau at Machache later, because he has business to attend to here.

Today's bus ride was gruesome, the bus packed with sweaty bodies, most of which smelled terrible, and the seats not big enough to contain my legs, so that I was gritting my teeth against cramps through most of the bumpy journey. To make things worse, the driver was drunk when we started, and became progressively drunker on gin as the ride progressed; on steep hills he kept messing up the gears of the crawling bus, sending us careening backwards.

It was also irritating that people kept staring at me as if I were some sort of escaped zoo animal; it is odd for a white man to ride the buses. Furthermore, the bus driver stops the bus every ten minutes to chat with friends who happen to be passing on the road, or jumps out and runs to the home of a friend in a nearby village to say 'hello'. By the time we got to Leribe, I was in a temper which I had barely been able to control during the trip in the noisy, hot, smelly, cramped, crawling, constantly stopping bus. A couple of stiff brandies in the hotel bar saved me from exploding. I still have New York nerves.

There was one lovely moment during the bus ride, while everyone was shouting and bumping about the crowded aisle. I felt something lightly touching my arm in a strange manner, and looking down I found a tiny child of about three leaning over my wrist, his ear pressed with fascination to my ticking watch.

Yesterday morning, all ready for the trip to Machache, I learned that contrary to what the doctor had told me, there are no jeeps running from Palamas; a bus does go to Palamas, a small village about halfway through the mountains to Machache, but there's no public transportation beyond that point. I therefore went to see the people who run privately owned Land Rovers into the mountains for diamond mining. The bosses were away, but I spoke with a pleasant man, English I thought, who said that whenever they send a jeep into the mountains it is full to the weight limit, and that they can't take passengers anyway because of the great danger involved in the trips. Rather discouraged, I figured that I would have to reregister at the hotel and take a bus to Palamas the next day—and then just hope some other sort of transport might come along.

Depressed about being stuck in this dusty, dead town of Leribe, I returned to the hotel to register for another night. The woman who runs the place, however, told me angrily when I arrived that two 'Africans' had come looking for me and had been rude to her. She was highly indignant. Instead of signing in for the night, I went out to check on who it might have been; I figured it must have been Mr. Mohau, and perhaps a friend of his, for no one else knows me here; it certainly would be out of his character, however, to be rude. Sure enough, when I left the hotel I found Mr. Mohau and a school teacher friend of his who told me that they had gone to the hotel office to ask for me, and that the woman had become indignant because they refused to treat her obsequiously. We spoke for a few minutes, but since I was exhausted, I suggested that they drop by and see me later in the evening.

When I got back to the hotel office I was told that I couldn't have a room unless I promised not to have any 'black visitors'. I went into a rage; I had been under the naïve impression that this kind of thing couldn't go on so blatantly within the British borders of Basutoland. I told the woman that I'd rather sleep in the street than patronize her damned segregated hotel, and assured her that the District Commissioner of Leribe would hear of this outrage.

Out on the pavement in front of the hotel, I met again the second teacher from Machache, and as we were talking about what had happened, the hotel proprietor came walking by us.

Though we were standing on the edge of a wide path, she yelled at the teacher, 'Don't you have any manners—haven't you been taught to step out of a lady's way when she passes?' The teacher just took it, mumbling something incoherent under his breath. I wasn't so subdued in my comment.

The teacher and I parted, and after having a drink, I found myself with my suitcase, portable typewriter, and cardboard box heavy with canned food rations—with no place to go for the night. Worried, not knowing where to turn, I decided to go back to the man I had spoken to earlier about jeeps into the mountains. I walked to his home, an hour's trip with my bulky load, the dust blinding me and leaving me gasping. I arrived in a desperate condition, upset and exhausted. Seeing me standing there looking helpless out in front of his building, he came out and said, 'Did you have any luck?' I answered, in a shaky voice, 'No, I'm in a mess. . . .' He laughed, and said, 'Did you have trouble at the hotel?' I told him the story, and he said that it happens all the time—so often that the local people who feel the way we do have formed a club and built their own unsegregated bar as an alternative to the hotel pub. They did this as a last resort, when the District Commissioner was unable to do anything about their complaints about the hotel's policy.

My newfound friend had only an army cot and a sleeping bag to offer me—but that was more than enough—and we set it up in an old hangar on the property. We ended up having a fine evening together, drinking and talking and listening on his radio to good music.

The next morning, I went back into town in hopes, wild hopes, of finding a ride all the way to Machache rather than just as far as Palamas. While I was sitting in the dust at the side of the road, my friend came driving up in a jeep to tell me that he had a truck going up to the mountains, and had made room in it for me. It was going past Palamas to a point about twelve miles from Machache, and would leave me on the road. We drove back to his place, loaded me and my baggage onto the truck, and off I went.

Though the ride in the jeep truck was a bit terrifying, a few of the turns so sharp that the driver had to back up three times, his rear wheels inches from cliff edges, it was also lovely. This part of the country appears almost sub-tropical; all along the trail were flowers coloured striking red, and a kind of lily of fine delicacy—small and wax-like, almost translucent. We passed a few small deer, or *letsa,* and saw many birds—birds of dark greens and iridescent greens, with beaks three inches long and huge, drooping tails; there were yellow Cape canaries and bright violet birds. Of course there were the usual swooping, menacing hawks and rock-sitting vultures.

It was three in the afternoon when the driver let me off on the side of the road. I picked up my load, and started walking—knowing very well that I'd never be able to travel the distance to the mission, but feeling the necessity to make some sort of effort. I must have travelled about three miles before my arms gave out; I could have cried out of frustration at my weakness. Already it was late in the afternoon, and still I was stranded in the middle of nowhere, not knowing where to turn, what to do.

I knew that I somehow had to beat the darkness, so, leaving my parcels under a bush near the track, I went on walking without them. Soon I came within sight of a not-too-distant village—if a cluster of three mud huts can be called a village—and walked off the track in that direction, down the side of the mountain. I was met at the huts by a man who stared at me incredulously, and shook his head dumbly when I asked whether he spoke any English, any at all. In that moment of urgency and despair, I found myself speaking Sesotho as I hadn't thought possible—words coming to my head that I hadn't realized were in my memory. I explained as best I could that I had to get to the Protestant mission at Machache, that I was about to collapse from exhaustion (words were hardly needed to convey that), and that I was badly in need of a horse. With reluctance, after ten long minutes of deliberation, the man agreed to lend me his horse, for a few shillings, with my agreeing to hire someone to return it to him the next day. Overwhelming him with thanks, I paid him and took his horse, riding it back to the jeep track and loading onto it my luggage. It was necessary to put my typewriter and suitcase in front of me on the saddle and to hang onto them as I rode, but the cans of food fitted into the saddle bags.

Dusk came down quickly, and I rode blind, trying every moment to fight down a tendency to panic; fortunately I was on the jeep track and thus had good odds of finding my way and not getting killed on rough trails. Nevertheless, the darkness was terrifying; it felt solid, pressing heavily and obstinately on my eyes, refusing to let them adjust to its thick blackness. I rode on in what I hoped to be the direction of the mission, surrounded by the roaring of mountain streams and the sound of crickets, swimming blindly through the night, which was thick as syrup. It was a strangely spiritual experience, yet full of dread.

At one point I passed two horsemen who were going by in the opposite direction. The night was so strange, so blinding to the eyes but loud to the ears, so full of sharp mountain sounds which are unnoticeable to the seeing, and yet so deadly silent at the same time, that it was impossible to shatter the stillness, to utter a greeting. They rode by wordlessly, like sleepy phantoms—leaving me unsure a moment later whether they had really been there.

I wanted to stop and wait until morning, but it was bitterly cold, and I had no way of tying the horse. My face and hands were becoming numb in the freezing air; I could hardly feel the reins in my swollen hands. I kept lighting cigarettes, for the glow gave me substance, assured me of a reality. When I heard a faint sound of voices singing in the distance I feared that my ears were deceiving me; soon I saw the glow of a light, far away, blurred and unstable so that I couldn't be sure of my senses. But then the lights became definite, and the singing clear—the most beautiful singing I've ever heard. An hour later I reached their source, the Protestant mission, and was led to the dispensary by the minister, the Reverend Mohale.

I was awakened at six this morning by a loud pounding on the door. When I dragged myself out of the sleeping bag and answered the knock, I found the Reverend Mohale standing there with the chief of the village; chief or no chief, I excused myself for half an hour to wash and dress. When I came out, in slightly better condition, I found that the people of the village had gathered with the chief to greet me; there were about fifty people and they expected me to speak to them. I spoke with them first about our hopes of building a hospital, the principle of self-help, and the importance of their working for themselves. It went over well, and they all enthusiastically answered together, 'We agree. We like what you say'. I asked directly about the apparent fear the people have of going to see the doctor. The chief answered, saying that men from the mission had passed a false petition and had sent it to the government saying that it proves the people don't want a doctor here. He says that everyone is angry about it, and that he has sent a messenger to the lowlands to try to locate the document. I explained to the people without rancour that Dr. van Aswegen had been told by the Catholic mission that no doctor is needed here since the mission has a clinic, but that the doctor, knowing the needs of the community, told the priest that he was going to continue practising if the people so desired, despite mission opposition. Finally I emphasized that we need their help and their trust in the doctor so that they can tell the people who have been made afraid by threats that they should have no fear of coming to the doctor. They received this with cheers, all throwing their hands up in the air and shouting affirmation. A few people made short speeches describing how they had been sick before the doctor's coming and saying that they spoke for everyone when they said that all should support the doctor and help themselves establish a hospital.

The *pitso*, or meeting, was a great success; there can be no doubt that the people are anxious to have a doctor's services—Dr. van Aswegen in particular, for he is clearly much respected and appreciated here.

After the meeting, young Mr. Mohale, the son of the minister and a highly educated man, rode with me to the Catholic mission to see the head priest. At the mission, we were met by a friendly Mosotho priest who indicated that Mr. Mohale should tie the horses and that I should follow him to the head priest's office. When I said that Mr. Mohale and I were here together to see the Father in Charge, the man looked at us with mild disapproval, and pointing out the head priest's office, left us alone together to take care of the horses.

The Father in Charge received us cordially; he was a pleasant-looking young man, of about twenty-eight, from Quebec. We spent some time making small talk. When he asked me where else I'd lived in the mountains, and when I told him Sehlabeng, he smiled, and referring to the priest at the Sehlabeng mission, asked 'And how is Der Fuehrer?' When we began to talk about the unfortunate reason for our visit to him today, he told us, with convincing sincerity, that he knew nothing about a petition. He went on to say that he would certainly not tell the people not to go to the doctor—that he would have no right to say such a thing without the permission of the bishop, and anyway, though he didn't know the doctor well, he was impressed with him and thought he was doing fine work.

When we left the mission we were a bit confused—for the priest had been convincing. After we had spoken to a few people back in the village, however, our scepticism increased. The first thing we found was that the two men of the village who had done the dirty work of passing the petition—the chief's son and a man named Motaka (who is a big shot in the Nationalist party, a conservative party virtually controlled by the Catholic Church) —had both left the village after the morning's meeting and hadn't returned. We also learned that the day before these two men had passed the petition around the village, Motaka had met with the priests at the mission and had refused to tell anyone what the meeting was about. For what it's worth, the general feeling among the villagers is that the chief's son is a pawn of the mission, that the priests have been trying to persuade the chief's son to have us kicked out of the village, that the priests are angry because since the doctor came the mission hospital has had no patients and therefore isn't making any money. All this is hearsay, highly unreliable, and we don't know what to think.

But one thing is sure: wherever I go in the village now, people tell me that the doctor must not stop coming—that they want him here very much and aren't listening to those who say they should not go to the doctor when they're sick.

Today the doctor came, and after talking over what had happened, we decided that the best thing to do is to go right on working whatever the attitude of the mission may be, since the people want our service and are behind us. With things regarding the mission so vague, we can only dare assume that the priests are speaking sincerely.

Our take-off from Machache airstrip brought us close to disaster. When we started our run down the strip there was no wind, but just as we were leaving the ground a huge cross-wind gust came from nowhere and blew us sharply to the side. Our right wing narrowly missed the wall of a hut, and we headed straight for a nearby mountainside—with the wind largely in control of the plane. In desperation, the doctor held the plane on course towards the mountain, hoping for an updraught to give us lift. He found it, and we skimmed over the rocks into safety. Before flying on, Dr. van Aswegen turned the plane towards the mission, and circled the giant cross they have erected on top of one of the mountains. Later he told me that in all his five hundred odd hours of flying, he's never come quite so close to getting killed—that he had flown over the mission cross to say a prayer of thanks. I remarked that I had thought he was cursing the priest for sending that gust our way. Laughing, he replied that he had been able to feel my anxiety on the seat behind him—that he had never seen anyone smoke so many cigarettes in one flight (never mind the No Smoking rule).

We flew to nearby Khubetsoana district, where the doctor intends to establish a hospital unit, and surveyed from the air the possible sites for building. The area has a remarkably dense population. Finally we landed at the village proper of Khubetsoana, where the dispenser, Molopo Moshoeshoe, has been stationed for some time, setting up a temporary clinic. We discussed with Moshoeshoe the matter of which village would be the best location for a hospital, and he told us that by our looking around, considering possibilities, we have created communal competition.

One day last week, seeing a village with a rather flat bit of ground nearby which could become an airstrip, the doctor landed his plane (the village was about three hours' horseback ride from Khubetsoana where the clinic is presently situated). Hundreds of people swarmed about him, and there was an on-the-spot *pitso* to discuss the possibilities of building a hospital. The people insisted that their village would be the best place, that they would all do everything in their power to help themselves build a hospital and run it. Later the same week, two other villages near Khubetsoana sent their chiefs to Masianokeng to see the doctor and suggest that he work in their villages. The next time he flew over their homes, the doctor found that the people of both communities had levelled airstrips so that he would be able to land. He landed at one, but the other was impossible: the people had lined their strip with huge boulders painted white, but since the strip was only about ten yards wide, the stones made landing dangerous. As he flew low over the strip, he could see the disappointment on the people's faces; how could they understand why he didn't land?

At Khubetsoana itself there is already the beginning of a clinic in a hut lent to BASOMED by a local family; as usual, patients requiring hospital treatment are given the use of other local huts. Since this village is nearly central to the area's population, and since we are already partially established here, this would probably be the best place to build. The airstrip is concave, becoming a small lake after rains, but we have an idea for a new airstrip location only a few hundred yards distant.

On Christmas Day, the doctor and I flew to his parents' farm near Bloemfontein. Carl (van Aswegen) told me before we left that he is anxious for me to meet his father—that I must try to understand him, and appreciate him for all that is good in him.

Mr. van Aswegen is a sturdy, hard Afrikaans farmer—an ardent Nationalist who fought the English in the Boer War. Any warmth he feels, he keeps hidden under a thick, cruel-looking crust; in the Afrikaans tradition, he wants to see his son Carl take over his farm when he dies, and it pains him deeply that instead of farming, his son is 'working with the damn *Kaffirs* in Basutoland'. He constantly makes cutting remarks about his son's working for nothing; he refuses to acknowledge that Carl is accomplishing anything, for 'if a man works, he gets paid for it!' As he and I walked around the farm, I battled with him, trying to get him to admit a pride in his son's work, but he stubbornly expressed nothing but disappointment and anger at his son's actions. At one point, he motioned toward a piece of farmland, and said, 'That's Carl's. We've put it aside for him, and it will be there for him whenever he decides to come home.' When I referred to the plot of land as a 'farm', the old man muttered bitterly, 'It isn't a farm. It's just a piece of useless land until my son comes to farm it.'

Mrs. van Aswegen, however, is one hundred per cent mother and backs Carl in his work, even coming to Masianokeng to help him at times. Despite the friction created by Carl's father's stubborn feelings, both his parents are so overwhelmingly considerate and kind deep down that it's wonderful to be near them. Meeting them helped me to understand Carl better, and gave me a deeper awareness of the struggle within him as he goes about his work. He's their only living child.

It was a nice Christmas, quiet and relaxing except that we

found ourselves still being battered by BASOMED problems. It isn't possible to get away from them.

Troubles at Masianokeng have mounted to such a point that we just feel constantly dizzy with ambitions, frustrations, and sometimes depressing hopelessness. First, we must concentrate on the work itself: we have £4000 donated by the Calouste Gulbenkian Foundation for capital expenditure in the establishment of mountain clinics. Some of that money has been used for the stocking of clinics, and with the rest we have bought material for ten prefabricated steel buildings with which to build two five-building hospital units. One unit will be central to the northern, Khubetsoana, area of the mountains, and the other hospital unit will be a central station for the southern, Sehlabeng, area of the mountains. We must decide definitely in which villages to establish these hospitals, and meanwhile people are crying that they want the hospital in their own village. Secondly, we find ourselves constantly being discouraged and diverted from the essential work by the fears, jealousies, and politics of missions, and hindered by the complete lack of government support. And thirdly, a recent letter has brought to its climax our destroying financial problem—forcing us to concentrate on the solution of a large debt. When the doctor established the organization BASOMED, he put all his personal savings into the effort; finding that still more money was needed, he preferred to run up a personal debt rather than see the people in need of medical service die. In order to protect BASOMED he took this responsibility in his own name. Now it appears that for all his effort and accomplishment, the reward will be personal ruin; the creditors are refusing to wait any longer. He owes a total of £8000. The BASOMED property is worth more than twice that amount, but that doesn't save the situation. We don't know what to do, except to beg the creditors to hold off a bit longer in the hope that we can somewhere, somehow scare up a grant.

Yesterday a woman came to the doctor in a state of shock. Her story was tragic, and horribly typical: her husband went to the mines in Johannesburg a number of years ago and never returned, leaving her with three sons, aged fourteen, sixteen and nineteen. A month ago, her two older boys went off to the Republic mines. (The younger of the two was by our records a serious tuberculosis suspect, but he nevertheless passed the Native Recruiting Corporation physical examination to work underground).) Just a couple of weeks after they started work, both were killed in a mine accident. The Native Recruiting Corporation informed the Basutoland government, the government informed the chief of the mother's village, and a few days later a messenger of the local chief walked into her hut and said, 'I have been instructed to tell you that your two sons are dead in the mines.' She doesn't even know how, when, or where they died, and has no information about whether or not they were buried. Now she's in a state of mental collapse, and both she and her surviving son are starving, for she is without means of living. We are doing all we can to help them, but we have no funds, and will probably get little or no co-operation from the Native Recruiting Corporation in our efforts to get information on the accident and locate the boys' clothes and other belongings.

What can we do?

These days with all their worries are so depressing, so many difficulties coming with each new day that we find it hard to meet the sunrise. As Carl and I sit outside in the late evenings discussing various pressing problems, hashing them over and over until a solution pops into our heads, new things keep appearing. While we were outside the other evening, little kids started coming to us asking for Christmas gifts; we gave them sweets, and they were all excited. One particularly bright fellow came over to us alone. The doctor asked whether he went to school, and the kid, about twelve years old, explained that he doesn't go to school because he doesn't see well. When we asked about his parents, he said that he hadn't seen his father for years and that his mother is out of the country—that he is living with friends here and there. So, despite all financial difficulties, we were forced to get him glasses, and he is now living here with Josepha and Sechlobi, helping around the house and gardens.

This individual case coming along during our discussion of overwhelming problems was no distraction—for the problem the boy had was no less relevant than any of the general topics we were worrying over. We are just trying to figure out how it can be possible to do something for him—for three hundred thousands of him; and while we try to do something positive for him, we are beaten down and discouraged by the realization that this boy's humanity is not recognized in full by either the optician who will eventually (with feelings of self-righteousness) sue us for the cost of the boy's glasses, or by all those people who stand apathetically watching this boy's misery. While they ignore the basic realities of human meanings, they will be scornfully calling us 'hopeless idealists'.

In going through the files on the doctor's desk the other day, I came across a football lottery card. When I asked Carl what this was doing here, he explained that he puts a small amount of money into the lottery every few months in the hope that BASOMED might win. Then he chuckled, laughing deep in his throat, a powerful stomach-shaking chuckle which appears to shake off all his problems for a moment before they return to overcome him again. Today we got a letter which read, 'Tough luck—you missed a £50,000 jackpot by only one number.' With it was a free lottery ticket for another try. It made us feel pretty lousy; all day we kept seeing mental pictures of what we could have done with £50,000 in these poverty-ridden mountains.

The doctor has been treating me so much as an equal, giving me so much responsibility and trust, that my inadequacy often worries me. The other night at dinner, I hesitantly told him that though I appreciate the tremendous responsibility he entrusts me with, he must be ready to correct my mistakes. I am perhaps too impulsive sometimes, among other things. He said that he often forgets how young I am, but that on Christmas afternoon at his parents' farm, when exhaustion overcame me and I fell asleep, he came into the room, and upon looking at me realized with guilt the burdens to which he was exposing me. But, after thinking for a moment, he made some remark about all people being just kids until they come to grips with things.

Sometimes I see him in a state of near collapse from exhaustion and constant discouragement, and I feel upset and sad that he's so alone with such a large burden; it's wrong that he should have to sacrifice and risk so much, and be so alone in doing it. These problems are not one man's problems—they are problems created by the negligence of men, and are not rightly to be left for recognition and solution by one man, or even two alone.

The other day when the doctor and I were talking with the

Khubetsoana dispenser, Molopo Moshoeshoe, about plans for building a hospital there, Molopo happened to ask me how long I would be in Basutoland, and Carl answered for me, 'A few years, at least.' I started, and told Carl that I can't promise more than a year's work here because I have obligations at home. Carl, upset, and effectively unreasonable, said, 'So, Mr. Moshoeshoe, we'll build a hospital at Khubetsoana and the people will have its services until next autumn. Is that okay?' I told him that he was being unreasonable; I was somewhat angered, but at the same time really troubled by the question of how, once involved, one can leave this work. Carl softened up, and said, 'Well, can't you get some other people to help? Somehow we must get help.' His voice became desperate—we need help. I asked him to please not press me too hard, told him that I feel as he does and, as he knows very well, am trying my damnedest to get help. It isn't easy. He saw that he had reached me, as was his intention, and boosted me now with, 'I'm sorry, but I want to see a Jeff Baker at every one of our clinics.'

I suppose the day will come when I'll have to leave, though doing so will leave me with no peace of mind. When it happens, for whatever reason, I'll be letting Carl down. This isn't a problem to be worried over now, and we both know it—but these are times of stress and loneliness. The doctor needs men to help him with the monstrous job he's undertaken, and as an individual he needs some support too.

I'm very worried about him. He's working far beyond one man's capacity, and the problems on his mind are an awful strain in themselves. This morning he flew Rosalia to Bloemfontein when she received news that her mother was dying. When he came home, I met him at the plane, and as he stepped out his hands were trembling. I tried to persuade him to take a rest, for his sake and for the sake of the people for whom he's providing such an important service. But he hates discussions forcing him to thoughts of himself and this makes it almost impossible for me to bring up the matter of his health and safety.

I have grown to love this man, not only for the good he accomplishes through highly-motivated and strong action, but also for what he represents. His very presence ennobles one. He is not a man one idolizes—he is a man one deeply appreciates. He is a man speaking through his actions, and hearing from others through their actions. With him, there's no room for insincerity.

He has a power, a hypnotizing energy, which everyone around him immediately senses; some like it, others fear it. Yet, he often seems lonely with other people, and their fearfully narrow outlooks on things discourage him. And at such times he grows even more discouraged over his own intolerance.

He loves animals and they respond to him excitedly and trustingly. It's remarkable, and almost mystical, to see their instinctive and immediate trust in his presence. His natural and complete communication with the mountain people is also beautiful to see.

Carl and I worked out a plan for the mountain clinics. We have in Maseru at this time the material for ten prefabricated steel hospital buildings; they were especially designed to weigh one thousand pounds apiece, and to have no parts longer than seven feet. Thus they can be flown to the chosen hospital sites in a single-engine Lockheed aircraft, one building per flight. Five buildings are at present being flown to Khubetsoana by charter plane, and then the other five will go to Sehlabeng. A professional builder, Molefi Thinyane and I will put them up with the help of local people. They are designed to go up fast—just a matter of fitting the prefabricated parts together by plan—and will be strong enough to easily withstand the wild winds of the mountains.

At present we have in the mountains only scattered medical services, but soon our work should be well organized and as effective as possible considering the difficult conditions involved. In the northern part of the mountains we have a well-equipped clinic at Machache, staffed with a full-time staff-nurse/midwife and dispenser, serving a potential 17,000 people who previously had to travel two days on foot to the nearest hospital; in the southern area we have an established, fully-equipped clinic at Mafisa, staffed with a full-time staff-nurse/midwife and two dispensers, serving a potential 29,000 people who previously had to travel three days on foot to the nearest hospital. In addition to the well-established units, the doctor has begun clinics (after landing his plane on rough plateaus and persuading the local people to help themselves and build airstrips) in the north at

Mohokare (population 19,000, nearest hospital one and a half days), and Likhoiting (population 26,000, nearest hospital a full day away), and in the south at Sehlabeng (population 7,000, nearest hospital one and a half days away). We have decided to build one of the prefabricated units in the north, somewhere in Khubetsoana which is a central spot, and the other in the south, somewhere at Sehlabeng which is central to that part. Then we will have three central bases, Masianokeng, Sehlabeng and Khubetsoana, with surrounding sub-clinics for the mountain centres. Each clinic will have highly qualified full-time staff, and hopefully the doctor can visit each clinic one day a week, later improving on that with radio units, and perhaps help from a second doctor.

As soon as we can get a few of the most pressing administrative problems off our backs, the doctor wants me to go to work managing the Khubetsoana operation and later the Sehlabeng operation, thus giving him a chance to concentrate on his doctoring and flying; flying in the mountains is hazardous enough without his being completely exhausted and constantly worried about various difficulties aside from his patients' problems.

We received yesterday afternoon a letter from the District Commissioner of Leribe saying that the Father in Charge of the Catholic mission at Machache has brought to the attention of the police commissioner the fact that a petition was signed by many people of the area demanding that the doctor leave. The whereabouts of the petition are unknown. We were livid, first of all at the priest's implying in this manner to the authorities that the local people want us out—without being able to actually present a petition or other proof—and second at the distinctly unfriendly tone of the District Commissioner's letter. We wrote back to the DC, demanding that he and the priest find said petition before making charges or reaching conclusions harmful to our work and the health of the local people. In addition we decided that we had better take immediate action to defend our work, despite our reluctance to take defensive measures.

We feel that we must arrange an interview with the top man, Mr. A. F. Giles, the Resident Commissioner of the country, to explain and clear up this matter before rumour destructive to our work should reach him. We feel it important anyway that the

Resident Commissioner take active interest in our work, as a service providing socio/medical aid in previously neglected areas of his country.

Yesterday afternoon while the doctor was seeing patients at the clinic and I was clearing up back correspondence, Joe Mapetla arrived. Joe is the son of the chief of Masianokeng, as well as a highly successful lawyer in Maseru and Chairman of the BASOMED committee. I spoke with him for a long time about the Machache petition, BASOMED's rapidly growing mountain programme, and finally my disgust at how little the BASOMED committee members are doing. Joe was shocked at the mission difficulties, surprised to see how the mountain work has grown, and somewhat offended at my frank attack on the committee.

Just then Carl came in with Mr. Khakhetla, the Minister of Health, who had come as a patient. We brought him over to a pinned wall map describing the locations of the country's medical services, and he was stupefied to note what it so graphically says: it shows with brutal clarity the fact that the government medical services are all but one in the lowlands around the Basutoland border, and that the mission hospitals are similarly distributed—leaving BASOMED clinics almost entirely alone in covering the remote mountain areas of 300,000 population. Then, while Carl stood back waiting for a possible explosion, and Joe frantically signalling me to be more tactful, I told Mr. Khakhetla in most direct terms the facts about government and mission medical services. I pointed out that mission clinics are in most cases being run by completely unqualified, unregistered staff yet are receiving government aid, while our clinics receive no government aid but only regular notices warning us that each of our nurses must be properly registered or our service will be closed down; I told him of the atrocities to be seen at Machache mission 'hospital'; I explained to him that right here in the hospital-crowded lowlands half the teeth Dr. van Aswegen has to extract are teeth broken by unqualified nurses at mission 'clinics', and that almost all of our terminal cases—patients who die on the examining table—are people who have been kept for months at unstaffed mission clinics, brought to the doctor only when they begin to suffer the convulsions of death. Then, as Mr. Khakhetla stood with his mouth agape, I told him of the priest at Sehlabeng having removed the windsock from the airstrip when he heard the doctor was coming, and of the petition passed among illiterates at Machache.

He was too stunned to be diplomatic or angry; he simply fled.

Carl and I are going ahead with arrangements to see Mr. A. F. Giles, the Resident Commissioner, and are requesting the presence of Dr. Clark, the Director of Health; Mr. Khakhetla, the Minister of Health; and Major Mathias, a power at Barclay's Bank as well as our head trustee. We want first of all to show the Resident Commissioner what BASOMED is presently accomplishing and what a massive job it will soon be doing in the mountains, and then to explain that we have come to defend our work and the people it serves, and to say that it is due time we received some moral material support from the Basutoland government. There is much suffering in this country. There are three hundred thousand people in these mountains who may not be so important statistically, and may be hidden from the eyes of visiting British officials, but who are nevertheless miserable and dying human beings deserving of recognition.

Before seeing Mr. Giles, I decided it would be a good idea to have a chat with the Roman Catholic Archbishop of Maseru. Mr. Khakhetla, the Minister of Health, who had again come to Masianokeng for Dr. van Aswegen's medical advice (I hope it's not his heart) reluctantly agreed to take me to Maseru and introduce me to the Archbishop. With a personal introduction, I trusted the interview would go more smoothly.

We drove to the Archbishop's house, and after introducing me quickly, Mr. Khakhetla went back to his office. I liked His Grace immediately, and dared to hope that a sincere approach and frank discussion of what's been going on would bring him to understanding and productive action. His Grace, Archbishop Emmanuel Mbathoana, is a large man, openly friendly, and delightfully informal, almost jolly. We had a cordial beginning to our meeting, for he has spent some time in New York City and enjoyed talking about the place with a native. We were interrupted briefly by a Canadian priest who came in, knelt as he kissed His Grace's hand, and spoke with him for a moment in French before bowing and departing backwards.

I then launched into the upsetting reason for my visit, telling him that I had come to discuss with him a most serious and distressing matter, and explaining our exact difficulties with the missions at Sehlabeng and Machache. He said that he had no idea such things were going on, and assured me that he would send a message to the priest at Sehlabeng, adding that I must see the bishop in Leribe district concerning the Machache difficulties. I was not to be put off; I whipped out a map, pointed out to him the extent of BASOMED's work, and explained that we are very busy trying to provide a socio-medical service for three hundred thousand people in the long-ignored Maloti Mountain regions, and cannot possibly spend our time trying to combat interference on the part of the missions. When I elaborated on the social and financial exploitation of the people taking place in some locations, and described the 'medical' work going on at mission 'hospitals', he looked genuinely disturbed.

Feeling rotten, I asked him desperately, 'Can't we get some co-operation?' I told him that we don't want trouble—that we're trying to accomplish something constructive and want, if not co-operation, at least to be left in peace to do our work. I added, 'Think of all that could be accomplished here medically if we could get some co-operation from the missions. We've tried to co-operate, but are only thwarted in our efforts for the people by the very priests who should be helping them.'

His Grace agreed, and said he would like us to send him reports about BASOMED's progress so that he can figure out ways to work together with us. He promised sincerely to look into the situations I described and try to do something about them.

He's the first African Archbishop of this country, and these are the people of his country who are suffering. Perhaps he understands how easily the people of his country are taken advantage of, and how often they are mistreated. Perhaps he'll do something.*

The next day, the doctor and I had our appointment with the Resident Commissioner, set for 3.30 in the afternoon. Since we

* Archbishop Mbathoana kept his promise; he spoke with the priests, and his efforts did have a noticeable effect in that we had no more mission difficulties at Sehlabeng and Machache. I regret to report that on September 19, 1966, at the age of 62, Archbishop Emmanuel Mbathoana died of a heart attack during an aeroplane flight between Bloemfontein and Johannesburg.

had to take the plane to Maseru for refuelling anyway, we decided to fly in for the interview. We got into our best clothes, which for me meant khakis pressed to look as much like slacks as possible, shoes polished to look presentable but with no heels and with blackened twine for laces, a tie filthy and crumpled, and a sports jacket shapeless and dusty. I had nothing better, and could only hope that my appearance would arouse either sympathy or good humour.

We were, as usual, late in getting started, and at 3.15 rushed out of the house and began pushing the plane to the top of the airstrip, across which was blowing a furious crosswind. Carl surveyed the strip, considered carefully, and lined up the plane with its nose pointing into the wind, facing up and across the strip. We figured that the head wind would give us a lift off the ground after only a short run.

We jumped into the plane, in a frenzy at being late to such an important interview; Carl gunned the engine, and we headed up and across the strip into the wind. It was only as we left the ground that we realized we had forgotten something—simply the fact that there was a telephone wire stretching from the dispensary building to the road, right in our path. Carl leaned into the stick, diving the plane under the wire, missing it by inches; our wheels slammed into the ground and we bounced into the sky, into flight, our teeth rattling from the impact. The doctor turned round and looked at me, his face like death; I just shut my eyes and gripped his shoulder for support. He commented later, 'You're a wonderful passenger. You never say anything, but get more and more silent.'

We landed delicately at Maseru, hoping fervently as we came in that the plane still had an undercarriage, and rushed to the office of the Resident Commissioner, arriving ten minutes late. We were both pale and shaky, dying for a drink, paralyzed with lingering shock. Outside the office we met all those who had been invited, plus Mr. Waddington, the Government Secretary, whom the Resident Commissioner had requested to join us; they were all wearing formal dress.

We all nodded and smiled at Mr. Giles who sat behind a shiny, long desk in a plush office. We began to seat ourselves. Seeing that there were no ashtrays near our seats, however, I said politely, 'Excuse me,' walked across the room to where there was a pile of ashtrays stacked on a table, and came back with one which I placed on the floor between the doctor and myself. I lit a cigarette, and sank luxuriously into its drugged relief. Mr. Giles made a few jokes which caused everyone to laugh courteously, then we got down to business.

Carl began to speak, beginning with the situation at Sehlabeng, but finding himself in a state of incoherence from the strain of the near flight disaster, blurted, 'Mr. Baker is our public relations man; I'll pass it over to him.' I caught in Carl's eye that familiar devilish gleam he acquires when letting fate take over, and plunged in. Tossing crippling tact and unctuous hypocrisy to the winds, I began to describe the affair of the windsock at Sehlabeng, hoping a candid approach would win the day, discarding futile efforts at diplomacy in this matter unfit for diplomatic handling. When I mentioned that Molefi, in a frantic effort to warn the pilot of the wind direction, had run down the airstrip with a streamer of toilet paper, everyone present chuckled nervously. Mr. Giles, however, gasped, and lifting himself to a half-standing position asked: 'Can you prove that the priest took that windsock down, young man?'

Before I could reply, he settled back in his chair, and said mildly, 'I think Dr. van Aswegen had better continue this story.' Carl said calmly that what I had said was quite correct. Mr. Giles intervened to say that this was the sort of matter that would best be discussed by us with Dr. Clark, the Director of Health, across the street.

Carl nodded, suppressing any bitterness, and after requesting that Mr. Giles give us just a few more minutes to show him on his wall map where the BASOMED clinics are located, said, 'Your Honour, would it be all right if we smoked?' At the moment, Mr. Khakhetla, the Minister of Health, who was sitting to the right of and slightly behind the Resident Commissioner, was puffing away on a cigarette, and I was just about to take another draw on my second. Pointing a finger at me, Mr. Giles commented, 'That young man has been smoking without my permission ever since he entered my office.' Being unaccustomed to formal meetings, and British Colonial protocol, it had never occurred to me that I shouldn't go ahead and smoke!

After the doctor had pointed out our clinics on the map, Mr. Giles then moved to usher us out of the room to Dr. Clark's office across the street. Outside, Carl requested that Major Mathias come with us to Dr. Clark's office, hoping that Major Mathias's presence would provide a sympathetic influence.

Entering Dr. Clark's office, we found ourselves before a large wall map, covered with brightly coloured pins. The mountains were littered with tacks indicating numerous clinics which exist only in the minds and statistics of government. For example, there was a button marking Mafisa as a 'Major Red Cross Unit'. Carl blandly informed Dr. Clark and Major Mathias, who is Red Cross Secretary, that we had last week flown the Major Red Cross Unit down to the lowlands in the Super Cub because with our clinic there, it can be used somewhere else. It was a first-aid kit placed in the hands of the local trader's wife, Helen West.

Carl requested permission to put pins in the map, signifying BASOMED clinics, to bring the map up-to-date, and Dr. Clark said of course that he should do so. While Carl began sticking in the flag pins we had prepared at Masianokeng, I sat with Major Mathias before Dr. Clark's desk, speaking with Clark. I continued the topic of government responsibility, expressing openly my horror at the state of the country's medical services and blaming that state on the fact that those people in positions to do something medically do not have the time to care about the people. Dr. Clark told me that his position limited him, that he'd like to do more about all the suffering, and that he knew very well of some of the things that went on. I blurted out, 'Oh, then you do know! But you're a doctor, aren't you? Don't you have a commitment there, as a doctor?' I must have been mad! Fortunately for us, however, Dr. Clark took a paternal attitude, nearly patting me on the head as he explained in effect that I didn't know all the facts of life: 'You'll learn some day, naïve idealistic child.'

Carl had by now finished his work at the map, and called for Dr. Clark's attention. He had stuck two of the brightest coloured and largest flags in each BASOMED clinic site. The distressed Clark asked, 'Why have you put two flags in each clinic?' Matter-of-factly, Carl explained, 'Oh, red and yellow are the BASOMED official colours.' We left the office with secret smiles.

As we walked, or rather half-ran, to the pub, I said to Carl, 'Doctor, I'm sorry if I screwed things up.' He touched my arm, and beaming said, 'Oh, I think it was a most successful afternoon.'

To my exclamation of surprise he answered, 'Why, for one thing, they now know that we mean business; for another, by indicating that he has more important things on his mind, Mr. Giles gave us the go-ahead to do whatever we please without his permission; and finally, I doubt that he'll easily forget about our work after this interview '

In a rollicking mood, we sat in the pub swallowing doubles. Joe Mapetla joined us, and as we hilariously told him the whole story he didn't know whether to laugh or cry. He finally laughed, with the help of another drink.

Having got Joe into one of his best and most easily persuadable moods, we started into the subject of how disgraceful it is that the committee members never visit the mountain clinics. Joe said, 'Oh, no! Don't look at me, I'm not going to fly with you into those mountains. I don't want to get eaten by savages, or killed in that aeroplane.' We assured him that if he's good, we'll see that the savages in the mountains don't fry him or use him for medicine, and insisted that he get used to flying this very evening. Carl proposed that I should drive Joe's Mercedes to his home at Masianokeng, while Joe should fly back with him.

We soon found ourselves drinking alone, though with undiminished glee.

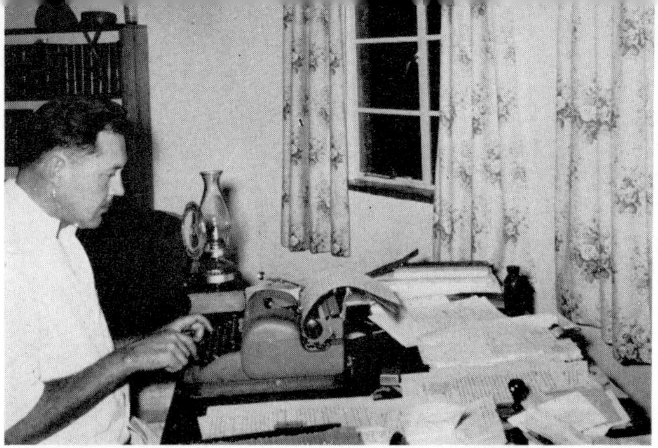

BELOW LEFT *Clinic building and dispensary, Masianokeng.*

BELOW *The doctors home and* BASOMED *headquarters, Masianokeng.*

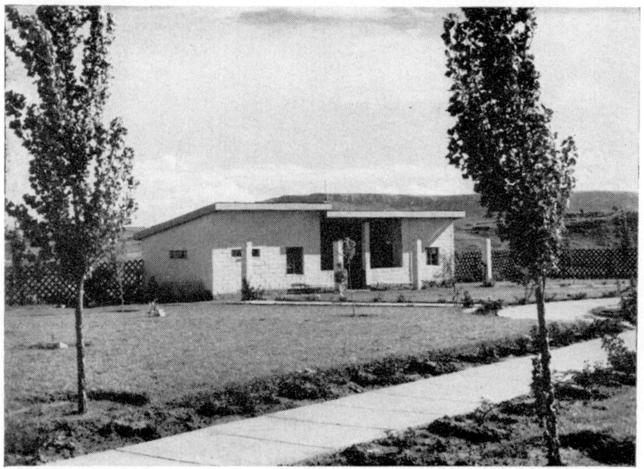

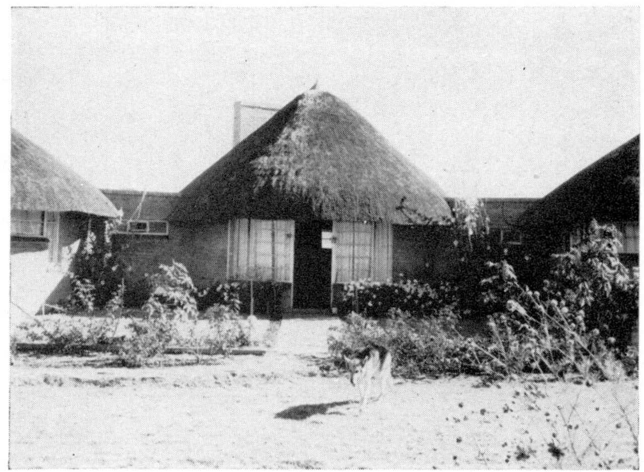

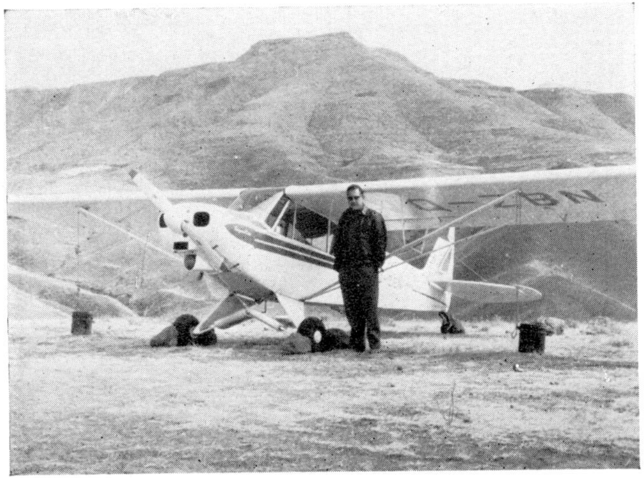

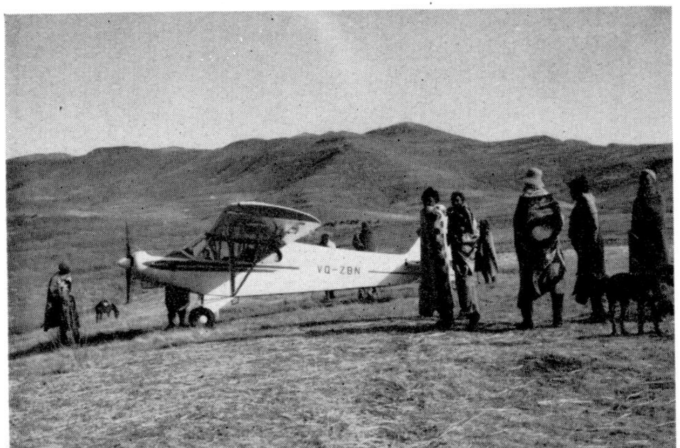

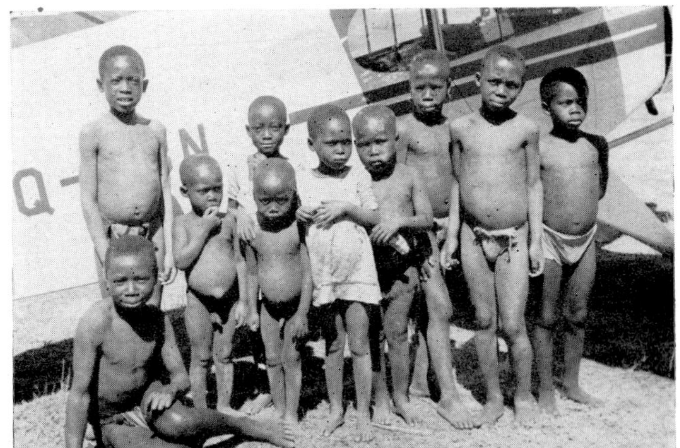

LEFT *Dr. van Aswegen by his plane.*

BELOW LEFT *Sehlabeng airstrip; 'Chief' is second from right.*

BELOW *Sehlabeng children.*

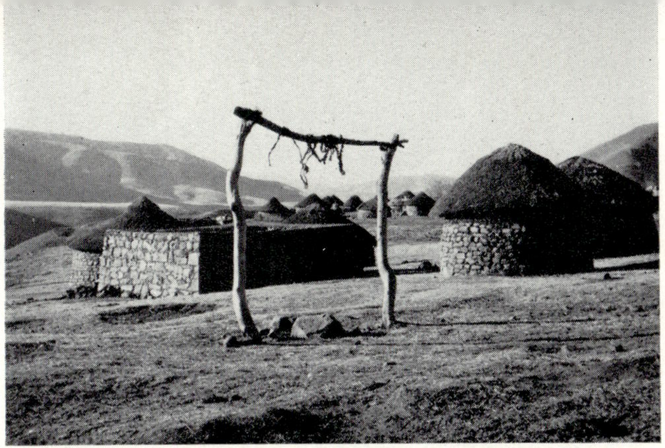

tanning rack for curing animal hides.

BELOW LEFT *A view of mountain flying — no room for error.*

BELOW *Molefi Thinyane and Jeff, Khubetsoana.*

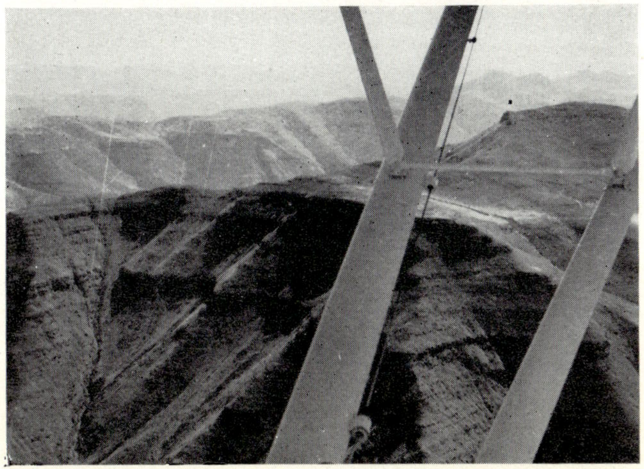

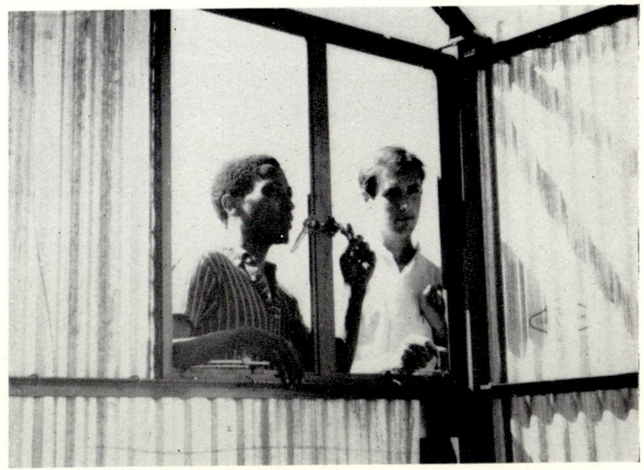

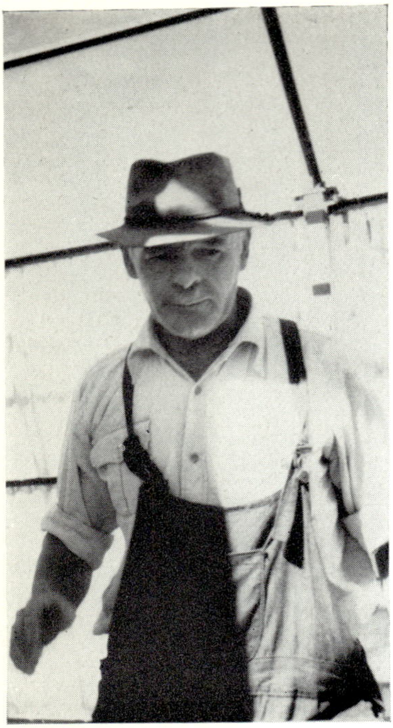

LEFT *Mr. van Jaarsveld.*

FIRST RIGHT *Stone wards for Khubetsoana Hospit*

SECOND RIGHT *A Picture of heal*

BELOW RIGHT *'Owc*

BELOW *The beginnings of a hospital.*

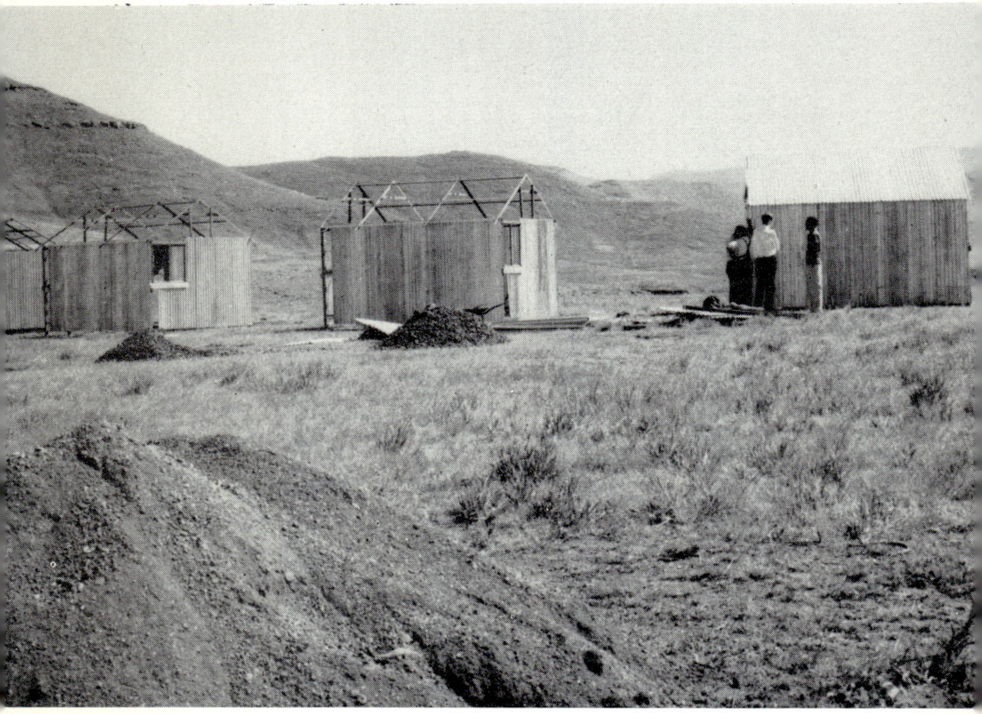

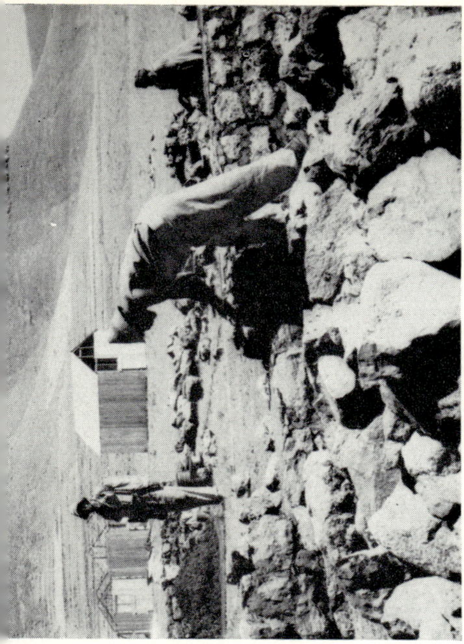

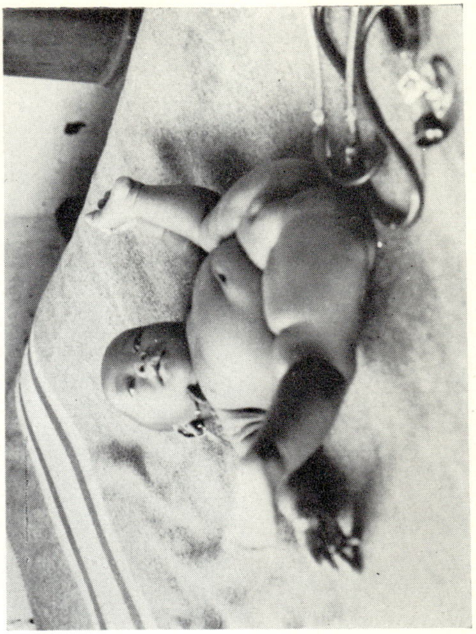

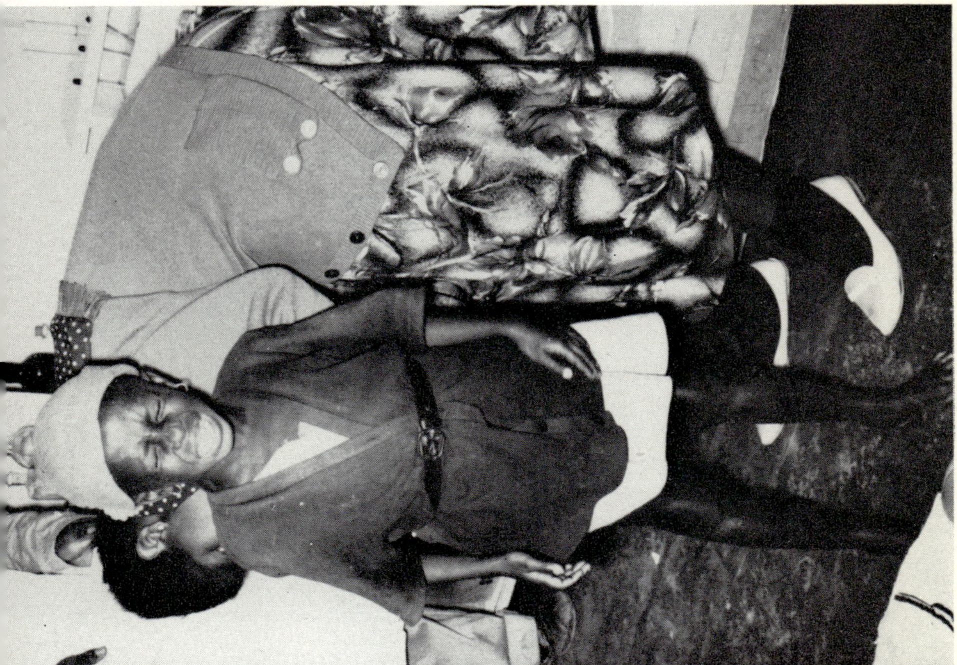

RIGHT *Youngsters dance, Masianokeng.*

BELOW RIGHT *Dr. van Aswegen examines a girl with cancer of the liver.*

BELOW *An aged patient, Masianokeng.*

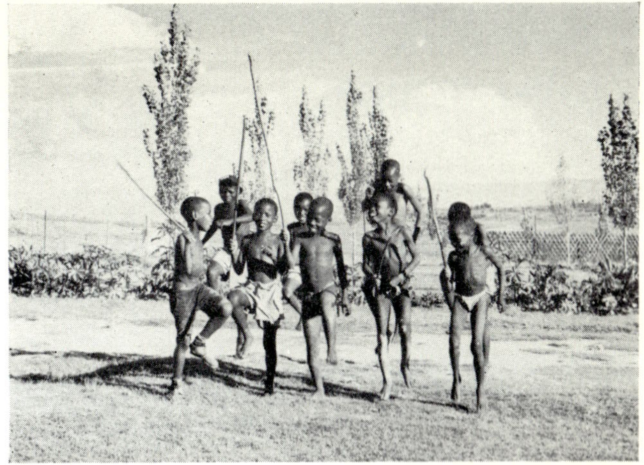

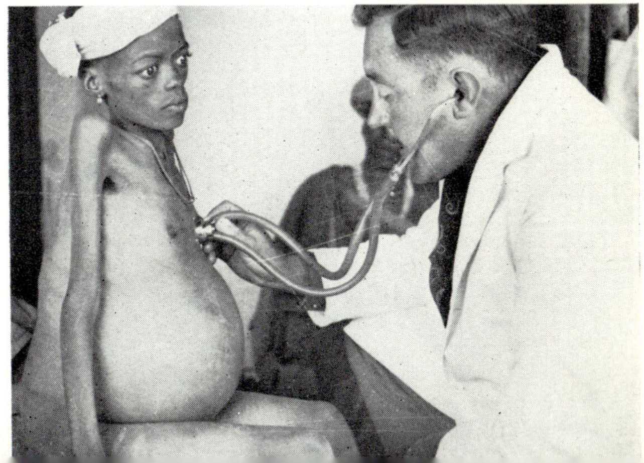

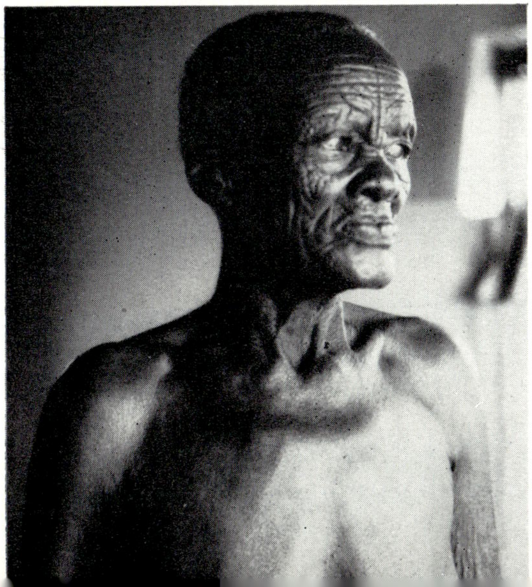

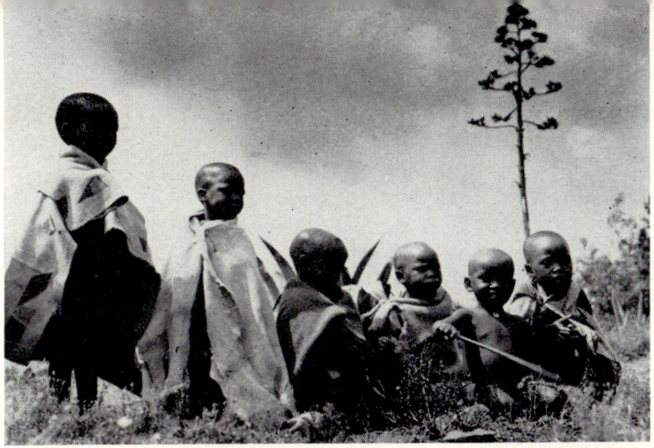

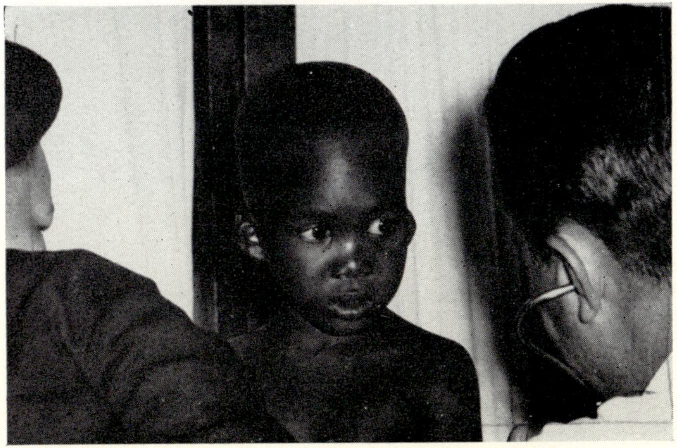

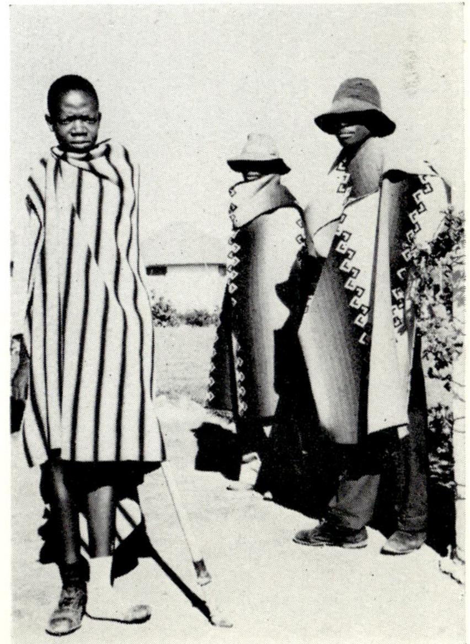

LEFT *These tiny children are herd-boys.*

BELOW LEFT *Dr. van Aswegen meets a young patient, Masianokeng.*

BELOW *Bethuel before treatment of tuberculosis, Masianokeng.*

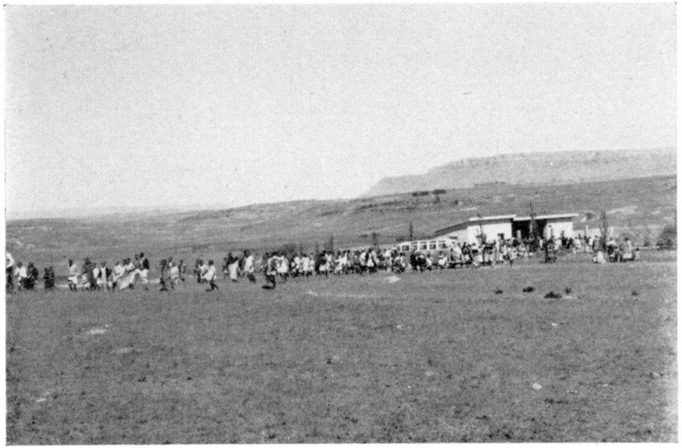

LEFT *Children swarm from the clinic after smallpox vaccination, Masianokeng.*

BELOW LEFT *The doctor is greeted by waiting patients at the airstrip, Masianokeng.*

BELOW CENTRE *In health, Basutoland is a country of beautiful people.*

BELOW RIGHT *Why must this young man face a barren future?*

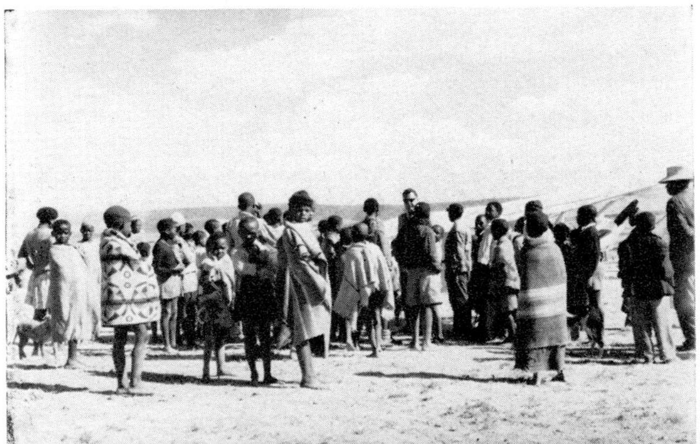

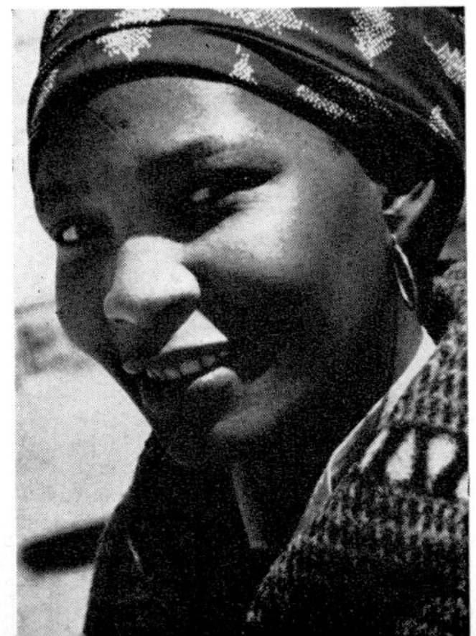

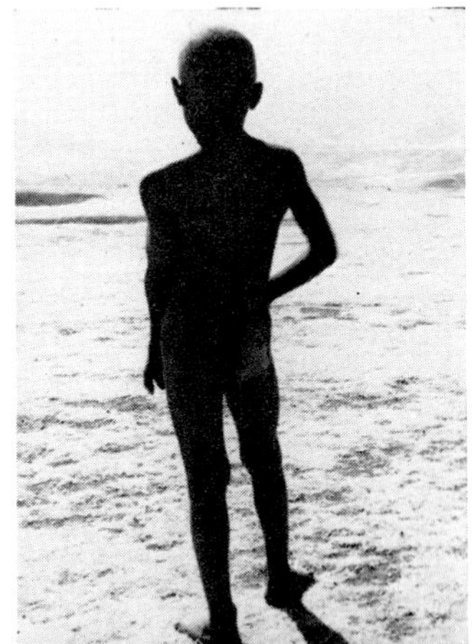

January 12 —February 20, 1963

The morning following the abortive government meeting was cloudy and the mountains were covered with mist, but we decided that we must try to reach the Khubetsoana clinic anyway, for we cannot wait any longer. Bad weather or not, we were determined to get back to our work with the local people, away from wasted time. When we got into the plane, we both felt uneasy—somehow we felt that something was wrong and didn't want to take off. We had to get there, however, and took off without incident, then faced the problem of getting over the escarpment, which was almost invisible in the mist. We searched around until we spotted a small opening into a valley through the clouds. One cannot allow his vision to be obstructed for a moment by cloud, for a few seconds of blindness can cause a crash into a mountainside; but we thought it possible to squeeze through this hole, which would bring us under the mist into a clear valley. From there it would be possible to fly up branching river valleys to our destination.

Nearly rubbing the mountainside with our wing-tips, we made it through the hole, and were pretty much in the clear—except for the fact that should a strong wind come up the valley we would be unable to get out unless lucky enough to discover another hole in the mist above us. We flew on, hoping for the best.

At Khubetsoana we found that the regular airstrip was thick with mud, as it always is after a rainy spell, being on concave ground. There is a plateau near by, however, where Carl has been considering levelling a multi-directional airfield, and there the ground looked fairly hard. Making a bumpy landing on the grassy plateau, after having swept over it a few times in search of rocks and anthills, we sank only a bit into the mud and met no hidden obstacles. It had been a hellish flight, and we just sat quietly by a stream for a few minutes to pull ourselves together.

Waiting for us at Khubetsoana was Molefi Thinyane, who had flown here a week or so before by charter plane; Molopo Moshoeshoe, who had come with him, was now in a nearby village where he had been called to a patient. While Molefi, the doctor and I looked around, trying to decide where would be the best place to build the hospital, we received a message from Moshoeshoe saying that a woman at the village of Phahameng had been in difficult labour for days and needed a doctor immediately.

Carl had recently established, with the help of the local people, a fairly decent airstrip at Phahameng, and now decided that he must fly there and transport the patient to a lowland hospital where she could if necessary be operated on.

We said goodbye, and he prepared for take-off. I felt worried, not only because of the poor condition of the strip, but also because so many things had been going wrong lately. I had an eerie feeling of danger. The plane came racing down the strip, into the steady head wind; Carl lifted it off the ground all right, just at the end of the plateau, and began to struggle to get out of, or over, a looming mountain before him. He didn't clear it by much.

It's a terrible thing to watch a difficult take-off; it's almost easier to be in the plane with Carl yourself than to have to stand by and watch him risk it alone. The day we went under the wire at Masianokeng, Moremi, a dispenser, watching from within the house, crawled under the bed and refused to come out for almost half an hour despite Rosalia's pleading with him. I know his fright, which must have been worse than ours though we were in the plane.

Molefi helped me get settled into the little hut where we will be staying until we get the buildings up. It is one of two huts belonging to a family in the village, and they have lent it to us voluntarily; meanwhile, the owner, his wife, and numerous children are all living together in their other hut next door. The clinic hut is similarly lent to us by another villager.

Many of the local people came to see who I was, and we spent some time speaking with them, until rain started to pour down and they dispersed. I was particularly happy to meet a man named Tsamai, a well-educated man who for unknown reasons came back to his home village in the primitive mountains after finishing a college education in the Republic; his father, who is away just now, is a famous herbalist, and thus the family is extremely rich. In contrast to the rest of this village of scattered mud rondavels, Tsamai has a fenced-in plot and numerous buildings of mud and stone, some of them square with corrugated-iron roofing. One of the buildings is called a shop, and another is marked 'Post Office', but both are empty and unused.

At dusk, while we were sitting in our crowded little hut, sheltered from a steady drizzle of rain but for a few leaks in the roof, I saw through the doorway a figure riding towards us from the distance. I was stricken immediately with the dreadful realization of my fears: it was a white man, his cheeks sunken, his face a bluish colour—he hardly looked alive. He rode up like a ghost. It was Carl.

We ran out, and he greeted us with a sickly attempt at a reassuring smile, making some remark about it being a lousy day for horseback riding. I looked hard at him; he nodded, and answered, 'The plane is wrecked.' He had come in as normal for a landing, testing the brakes per standard procedure, but when he touched down and hit the brakes they failed. The plane careened towards the river, Carl helpless to stop it, and by miraculous luck a rock about ten feet from the cliff edge stopped the plane, throwing it on its nose. As Moshoeshoe later described it: 'I saw the plane coming in as normal, but then it didn't slow down. It just kept going, past the end of the strip. I started running—I saw that it was going to go over the cliff into the river. But suddenly it went onto its nose, just before the cliff edge; the windows and roof shattered, and petrol pouring all over the place from one of the wings.' Moshoeshoe had run up crying, and helped Carl scramble from the plane. The petrol, thank goodness, didn't ignite.

Carl was a mess; we tried to relax him, and Molefi—a true genius—went out into the village in search of black-market brandy. Carl told us that the chief himself of the village of Phahameng had gone off immediately, riding furiously, to Sebesong six to eight hours away where there is a mission with a radio unit. He himself had borrowed a horse and headed back to us, but it had started raining, the shock of all that had happened had begun to affect him, and the horse he was on had come to a river and refused to move further. He had sat by the riverside in the rain for an hour, not having the heart to beat the horse into moving—these local animals are very badly trained—until finally a herdboy came along with some horses and agreed to let Carl borrow one of them to get here. He told us how, as he had sat there by the river, soaking wet, cold, discouraged, he had watched a scarab beetle struggle to roll a huge ball of dung up a small hill, failing again and again. He was a mess, unable to imagine ever flying again, wondering why he had ever begun trying to do the impossible.

Finally Molefi turned up with the brandy, and we bundled Carl off to a bed at Tsamai's house, leaving the bottle with him. We sat around hopelessly all evening. If lack of help, lack of funds, political and mission troubles don't make all of Carl's efforts useless, he'll be stopped by killing himself from exhaustion.

This morning Carl and I had a long talk; last night he felt that he never wanted to fly again; today he is finally convinced that he must not work himself beyond human endurance while at the same time carrying on a heavy flying schedule. In that respect, this accident may have been a blessing. He had wanted to work seven days a week, flying each morning to another clinic. Often he has talked to me about the necessity for an idealist to recognize the realities around him; now I told him that if he really believes in that necessity, he must recognize the limits of human endurance. We figured out a plan which would involve his serving for extended periods of time the three main clinics: Masianokeng, Khubetsoana, and Sehlabeng. One week he would fly to Khubetsoana, do clinics for four days, fly back to Masianokeng, and do clinics for three days; the next week he would fly to Sehlabeng, do clinics for four days, fly to Masianokeng, do clinics for three days. While at Masianokeng, since there are other medical services in the area, he could find time to rest. Perhaps, since Mafisa is near Sehlabeng, and is a comparatively safe strip, he could spend a day there also during the Sehlabeng week; it would be nearly impossible to give up that clinic because it is so well established. As far as other clinics go, those clinics which surround the centres of Khubetsoana and Sehlabeng each would have a resident Staff-Nurse/Midwife and dispenser; we can set up a weekly donkey-communication link between those subclinics and Mantsonyane at the end of the Mountain Road, and thus keep them in supplies. If the Native Recruiting Corporation comes through with the grant for radio units, those clinics can be in constant touch with the doctor.

Such a service, though not so impressive on paper, would be better for everyone in that it would have some permanency, and could run on a reliable schedule (weather would never allow a clinic-per-day plan to function smoothly). This way we would be providing a service which would not die a sudden death any day. Carl is an excellent pilot, but the best pilot in the world cannot live against a law of averages which promises death to anyone flying his previous schedule. Perhaps this near end will be the beginning of a more solid, lasting service.

It is two days since the accident. Yesterday morning the rain continued, making the airstrip impossible for the Maseru charter planes to land on. Hopefully they received the message which the Chief of Phahameng carried to the mission radio at Sebesong. We're very distressed because everyone at Masianokeng will be in a panic. Carl's parents will worry needlessly when they hear that Carl is missing, and every day lost means further delay in our medical service. Right now people at other clinics are gathered in expectancy of the doctor's arrival, many of them having ridden for days to reach him. They won't know he isn't coming until we can have charter planes drop messages to the clinics, and they won't have a doctor until we can make arrangements for our crippled plane to be towed out of the mountains and repaired.

While the rain poured down in the morning, Carl saw patients, and Molefi and I dispensed. Later, when the weather cleared, we searched for a building site. We worked harder than ever, trying desperately to convince ourselves that we can and must continue undiscouraged. I don't want to describe the full day and evening; we've been in a bad state. We went to sleep early, a restless night for everyone.

This morning we again worked extra hard, the doctor seeing

a heavy flow of patients, Molefi dispensing, and I at the chosen site. The weather has been perfectly clear, and the airstrip should be quite dry by this afternoon. Certainly a charter pilot could land and fly the doctor out, but we know better than to expect them to make a special effort. One would think they would try to do something—if not land with their Cub, at least drop some cigarettes and brandy.

We sat around and ate lunch silently. Just as we were finishing, a man arrived from Sebesong with a note from the wife of the trader. She wrote that the chief of Phahameng had arrived late at night with the message, and had gone to the mission where there is a large radio unit. The Father in Charge had come to the door, and when Chief Phahameng said that Dr. van Aswegen's plane had crashed and that he had an emergency message, the priest snapped, 'We don't take messages at night ' slamming the door. The chief had gone to the trader, and the trader, who has a small radio unit, had sent the message to the lowlands. I sent a note to the trader thanking him, and asking him to please get a message to the charter service to try to fly us out. I explained that the airstrip here is dry enough to easily accommodate them.

To describe Khubetsoana and the whole area: Khubetsoana is a fairly large village central to the northern part of the mountains, untouched by medical or social service. Khubetsoana village has the airstrip, which is basin shaped, flooding easily, and therefore unusable. We now have found a plateau nearby on which to build a more functional airstrip, and have located across a stream from that a large peninsula of land for our hospital. Chief Thaba of Khubetsoana has offered for our use that whole area of land, which includes two strong fountains, and a fairly powerful stream.

This is a densely populated area; the people in each village (Mohokare, Machache, Likhoiting, Phahameng) have been fighting for us to build the hospital near them. At one place, the local people levelled an airstrip in half a day so that the doctor could land there immediately; at another, the people built a strip and offered us numerous huts for hospital buildings and staff accommodation; at yet another, the people donated money at a community gathering, to be used for starting the hospital. Here at Khubetsoana this large piece of land with its fountains, which we have been offered, is large enough for a community farm, hospital buildings, and an all-directional airstrip; and it is surrounded by a stream so that we would have water if the fountains were to dry up. It is an exceptionally pretty site, and, best of all, it is central to all of the villages.

We have therefore chosen to build here; the surrounding villages at which people are willing to help themselves establish and support medical services will become sub-clinics. People in these surrounding villages can reach this main unit by horse in two to seven hours if necessary; in most cases the nurse at each clinic is qualified to treat them. In emergencies, a messenger can be sent to the doctor at the main hospital unit (in the absence of radios) and the doctor can fly to the sub-clinics.

As you stand on the hospital plateau facing north, you look up a great valley towards the river; facing east or west you confront huge mountains with rushing streams at their bases; and looking south you see another end of the valley, its flanks covered with groups of villages. Our scheme is to build a semicircle of five prefabricated buildings, facing north because of wind conditions. Other buildings to be erected immediately are stone wards which we will terrace off at an angle behind the semicircle.

Presently we are living within the village of Khubetsoana, about twenty minutes walk from the site. I sleep in a small rondavel lent to BASOMED by a family who own two such huts, Moshoeshoe sleeps in the dispensary, and Molefi sleeps all over the village, depending on where the party is. Carl is temporarily staying in a rondavel owned by Tsamai, and has himself become the happy home of five thousand hungry fleas. The rondavel where I sleep is everyone's kitchen, dining room, and sitting room; privacy exists only in my dreams.

This village is very different from Sehlabeng. At Sehlabeng we saw only the primitive, the poverty-stricken; here we see a startling blend of the primitive and the comparatively modern, the poor and the relatively wealthy. Here at Khubetsoana, where there is no mission near by, the people seem to have cultivated a bit of self-initiative. Many of them are quite well off, owning two or even three rondavels, some with tin roofs, windows and doors. Tsamai, of course, has the empty post-office building. And there is a man a couple of hours away who has had the initiative to get brandy from the lowlands and sell it here at black-market prices. Yet, with all this, there are people who are just as primitive and poor as those at Sehlabeng, people who live oblivious to all progress. Even those who have progressed go just so far and then stop; Tsamai, for example, with his comfortable buildings and university education, still has no chimney, and warms his home with a dung fire in the middle of the floor, choking off the air with smoke. Perhaps the smoky air reminds him nostalgically of his years in the city.

In the afternoon of the second day after the accident we laid out the building plan with nails and string, then arranged for sand to be brought by donkey from the river for making concrete; rocks to be dug, broken and dragged by oxen to the area for making foundations; builders to be found for constructing extra stone-building wards; small rocks to be gathered by children for the mixing of rougher cement for the floors. Much of the material for the prefabricated buildings is now in the village proper, the rest still to be flown up by chartered plane.

The next morning, local people joined us in the tedious and back-breaking job of carrying the steel prefab parts along muddy trails from the village to the site. Women and children hoisted heavy steel beams onto their heads, balancing them with incredible precision, and marched with seeming effortlessness towards the site. Molefi and I hoisted the beams to our heads, then tried shoulders, and finally just carried them along haphazardly, shifting the weight from muscle to muscle until we had no new muscles to shift to. The women, carrying the burdens of steel on their heads, paraded silently and expressionlessly; the children, carrying slightly lighter hunks of metal, sang as they went towards the site, and returned for more loads with wild dancing and bright songs. As they passed grazing donkeys, they joined hands and danced around the unsuspecting, sleepy-eared beasts until the poor animals hee-hawed in confusion and bewilderment.

After two trips, while the women continued to work, with no sign of stopping for rest, and the children appeared to be just gaining momentum, Molefi and I shamefully dropped with exhaustion. We could hardly remain standing; our bodies, now rubbery weak, threatened to collapse if we continued.

We found many other children, and told them that if they would gather small stones for concrete we would give them school exercise books and pencils. They were excited by our bribe, and ran about all the rest of the day making a game of collecting rocks into a growing pile.

After some persuading, a few men with donkeys volunteered to break and haul stones for the building foundations, and went to work. Chief Thaba himself volunteered numerous donkeys to be used for carrying bags of sand from the distant river. With all going so well, a builder showed up; his is a skilled job, requiring training and experience in building with stone. He really gave us a hard time, wanting a great deal of money for his work of building hospital wards. I explained to him that this money was not ours, but belonged to his people as would the hospital. But he was a stubborn bastard. Finally I told him to beat it, saying that he was being not only selfish, but a fool since this was only the first of many such buildings to be put up by the man who would work for a fair wage. We shouldn't have to pay him anything, but are willing to lay out a capital expense and pay him a moderate salary, because we know that he can't afford to work for nothing; but that he should demand ridiculous prices, as if he were bargaining with some trader who wants a building erected for his own profit, is too much even to listen to.

This morning I went early to the site while everyone else slept, and put the building materials in order. The people soon came to work, and Molefi and I again helped carry things until ready to drop. After some lunch, Carl, who had been seeing patients all morning, decided to go and lie beside a stream somewhere. He's badly in need not only of rest, but of privacy and a chance to think; he needs a few moments of peace, and had hopes of finding it in the quietude of the mountain valleys.

Soon, however, a rider came with a message from Molopo. The afternoon of the accident, Carl had flown to Phahameng to see a woman having difficult labour. Moshoeshoe now wrote from Phahameng that she had the baby all right, but has a badly torn vagina. We had to find the doctor, and no one knew where to look. We set off in different directions, climbing up and down mountainsides, searching along streams, climbing cliffs; finally I had to give up, and arrived back at the hut in a condition of such exhaustion that my legs were wobbling and I could hardly breathe. Climbing mountains at 8,000 feet is no easy trick, especially for a person who has never bothered with physical conditioning, and who chain-smokes green Basuto tobacco. Molefi came in to join me, and said that all was OK, he had found the doctor; Carl rode off to Phahameng to see the patient.

While searching for the doctor, I was down by the stream for a long while. The people of the mountains live high on the mountainsides rather than deep in the valleys because when they came to Basutoland they were in retreat of war and naturally took up defensive positions; to this day, they never build near a river, and thus get none of the benefit of lush ground and high-protein fish diet. The barren mountainsides on which the villages are situated have a desolate beauty of their own, but the rich loveliness of the land by the river is overwhelming. One is the mystical beauty of barrenness, the other the loud and colourful beauty of violently alive life: lush grasses as tall as a man, sweet and delicate flowers; the stream rushing in rapids after the rain, each jutting rock creating a small waterfall; the vegetation of the rich earth holding hundreds of birds in its paradise. Iridescent green birds, and black and red birds with long beaks and tails drooping a foot behind their small bodies. They glide along using their tails as rudders, or flap the tails slowly up and down, enabling themselves to hover over one spot, stopping time in its beautiful moment. Deep in a valley, looking around, all one sees is mountainsides; it's as if there were no people, no troubles, for miles and miles.

Back at the village, I anticipated another depressing evening and could not stand the idea. I wanted to get a bottle of brandy despite the excessive black-market price, but I had no money. But later, as we were cooking dinner, Carl produced a bottle as a surprise for us, and we poured out drinks into our enamel coffee mugs, turned on the radio to some static-full African jazz from Rhodesia, and began to feel some spirit. It was just what we needed; we were able to joke about all that had happened, to see it as an incident of the past, not of all time.

Today is again a clear day; if the weather would now hold until tomorrow morning the airstrip will be perfectly dry. It's Sunday, so no one is working. There is good music—Bach, Vivaldi, Mozart—on the South African radio station, and it is just right. As we sit listening to the music, some women come and sit quietly with us. They enjoy the music, becoming vaguely involved in it once they are over their wonder and fright at the radio. They accept the radio as part of us, whose strangeness they have accepted as we have accepted theirs; the music brings us all together.

Everywhere around the village one can see young herdboys playing an instrument called a *lesubi*—a long stick with a wire stretched along its length and a chicken feather for a reed at one end of the wire. When a boy hums on the quill, it vibrates the string and makes an eerie hollow-toned music. When the herdboys return at evening, each puts his animals in the kraal with the other animals of the village; in the morning each herdboy goes to the kraal, plays a certain tune on his instrument, and all his own cows, sheep, horses and goats come filing out while the others stay behind. Then he throws rocks at his animals and herds them off to graze on the barren dirt of the mountainsides.

Late in the day I spoke with four local builders about getting up the hospital wards. Three of them kept insisting on high pay. They see the aeroplane, our clothes, the typewriter, the radio, and think we have thousands of pounds to give away. They won't listen to reason, won't believe that we do not have funds, and cannot understand differences in standards of values between their society and ours. Finally one of the men, who had before said nothing, said that he understood that we don't have money, that anyway the people must help themselves rather than have money given to them, and that whatever money a builder is paid is money belonging to other villagers. He agreed to do the building for us at a cost of eighteen pounds including roofing, hauling of stones, and everything. Fine. Later, one of the men who had been giving us a hard time, came back and said that he would like a job hauling stones. We told him that he should go to the builder we just hired, since it is now his responsibility to hire men to work under him, paying them from the wages we are giving him for the total job. He complained that the builder would not pay him enough—but we were out of sympathy.

A plane came this morning, thank goodness, and took Carl and me back to the lowlands. Carl told me that he expects the problems there have been building up and therefore thinks it best that I come with him, returning to Khubetsoana later with the builder of the prefabs.

The mechanic, who came with the plane which flew us out, rode to Phahameng to see our Cub; he says that the aeroplane isn't too badly damaged—approximately two hundred and fifty pounds' worth, including a new prop which alone will cost one hundred pounds. With a temporary prop put on at the scene of the accident it can be flown out, and then the wing which is slightly bent can be straightened in the Republic. Good news of a sort.

We find our financial situation is more desperate than ever, our creditors really pressing, but it seems that a semi-personal letter I wrote to Mr. Betts of the Oxford Committee for Famine Relief explaining our position is provoking promising results. One of the committee members who is solidly behind Carl went independently to speak with Mr. Betts about our financial condition, and Betts expressed great concern and a willingness to help. He asked a couple of questions, however, such as, "Is it true that Dr. van Aswegen handles all money himself without anyone checking on him?' and 'Why is Jeff Baker called a volunteer worker when he is paid a salary of thirty pounds a month?' As for the first question, Carl never handles BASOMED money from patients, but rather leaves that to the dispensers at each clinic; outside donations are immediately put in the hands of BASOMED trustees in Maseru, and are carefully accounted for. As for Mr. Betts's second question, of course only my measly living expenses are taken care of by BASOMED, and they are much more than covered by the few funds I bring in from America. A discussion of our work with Mr. Betts should clarify things considerably. If he and OXFAM won't help us now, as they once did in donating the aeroplane, all the determination in the world won't keep the doctor's work alive.

There is a youngster of about fifteen staying with us, more as Carl's son than as a patient. His name is Bethuel, and he is severely crippled—unable to put his weight on one leg because of a pain in his hip. Carl wasn't sure what was the exact trouble with him, so he sent him to Bloemfontein to see a well-known radiologist. The X-rays we received indicate that Bethuel is suffering from tuberculosis—not of the hip, but of the spine. The difficulty he has with his hip is probably a transference of his spinal pain.

The damage already done is not great, but Bethuel will probably have to be completely immobilized in a cast for six months to a year—a torture for anyone, especially a young man his age, to go through. The doctors are not sure, however, that it is absolutely necessary to immobilize him; this is more than a clinical problem—it is a psychological one as well.

Bethuel has indicated to us that he once spent a long time in Maseru hospital, though he does not know exactly how long, and says he was put in a cast so that he couldn't move his legs. We decided this morning that I'd better go to the hospital and find out the details of his past treatment. Carl cannot hope to get any information there.

When I arrived at the British government hospital I was told by a doctor, 'It is certainly not possible to locate his records.' This was a bit beyond my belief, for in a hospital of this one's size and cost there must be at least some record of patients. I persisted, building up quite some unpopularity despite my forced friendliness, and was sent from one doctor to another—who doubtless thought me a nuisance when they were busy.

I finally made a Dr. Malcolm so impatient with my polite insistence, that he took me to the office of the matron, which I had not been allowed to enter previously. I was allowed to look through the hospital archives. After no less than an hour of searching through dust-laden, disorganized books, I found the boy's name and date of hospitalization. The matron told me, 'This is the only information available on the patient.' I answered, shocked, 'Do you mean to say that it's possible to find only a past tuberculosis patient's name and the dates of his stay in the hospital, nothing more?' I pressed her, insisting that this is a young man whose next year and perhaps whole life depends on our finding more information; finally she suggested that I speak with the doctor in charge of the tuberculosis ward who might remember Bethuel since the boy was there only a few months ago.

I found Dr. Rice, and asked him about the boy. He told me that he could not remember him. None of the nurses remembered the boy either. I was about to give up in despair, but decided instead to find out just what happens to a patient's records. The first nurse I questioned with 'Could you please show me the way to the room where the patients' records are filed' was very kind—

a girl of about twenty-one, a Mosotho. She told me as we walked to the room that she was a student nurse.

She took me into a dark and dusty room six feet by ten feet, three of the four walls lined with shelves. From floor to ceiling, bundled tightly on the shelves, and covered with grit, were ribbon-tied stacks of record sheets—in no order whatsoever. I felt like yelling with frustration and anger, that a hospital—and one built and run at such a great cost as this one—could care so little about patients as to keep no organized records.

At least, however, I had now located the records, and I'd be damned if I would leave without information about Bethuel's case. To the surprise of the nurse, I pulled a stack of sheets from a top shelf, standing on a chair to reach them, and began untying the ribbon to start the search. She said, 'Are you really going to try to find the boy's records?' I said, 'Yes, and I'm not leaving until I've found them.' She smiled, and said that she was supposed to be at class, but that she would now skip it and spend the day searching with me. She insisted, suggesting that we could thus cut the time in half, from a month to only two weeks of searching.

In fact we could have searched for a month had luck been against our efforts, but as it turned out, after only six hours of leafing through the rubble, we found Bethuel's two sheets. I read them, finding that the boy had been nine months in a cast. Although he had been treated for tuberculosis of the hip, I could find no record that any X-rays had been taken to check on his condition.

I copied the records for Carl, and thanking the nurse most warmly for her wonderful help, left for Masianokeng. Bethuel's problem is really depressing—Carl wondering how to tell the boy that he will have to go back into a cast (though not at Maseru hospital again). To think that there are thousands of people in this small country who are walking about with severe cases of tuberculosis until an abscess develops and they become progressively more deformed and weak until they just die in agony. Somehow the mass problem seems not a trifle more important than the case of just this one fellow.

For the past few days, having no aeroplane, we've mainly been feeling discouraged and sort of waiting for the OXFAM meeting Wednesday—or for anything good to happen. Today, tired of waiting and fearing that we may be waiting for nothing, I wrote nine long letters to various assistance-giving organizations in America whom we had not before approached.

Yesterday evening Carl told me with much determination that he has decided to do all the clinics despite the impossibility of it. He knows it is nearly suicide, but I couldn't change his mind. I can hardly argue with him strongly about it, knowing so well how he feels about the people's need for medical service. We can just hope that it will be a temporary arrangement and that we will soon get a doctor to help Carl and a pilot to take care of the flying. It's impossible—the whole problem here seems impossible.

This morning at the dispensary, Carl came across a discrepancy in a patient's records, and after investigation found that the receipts had been tampered with. Upon asking the patient a few questions and looking into the books, he discovered that one of his particularly dedicated dispensers—an older man—had stolen five shillings, making out a false receipt. Carl called the man into the examining room, and asked him a number of questions about the act, but he denied everything, making up many ridiculously weak and conflicting excuses. Disgusted with him, Carl gave up.

In the evening, the dispenser came to the house to see the doctor, and said, 'Doctor, I'm sorry I had to lie to you today; I wanted to tell you the truth, but Moremi (another dispenser) was there, and he being many years my junior I couldn't let him know that I had stolen.' Carl said to him, 'Now, Mr. Takele, give it to me straight—tell me what's going on.' Mr. Takele jumped to attention, looked Carl straight in the eye, and said crisply, with dignity, 'Sir, I stole five shillings.'

We're running into an unusual problem in the mountains as our programme is about to go into full swing. Up until now, the patients have been told by the dispensers, 'Please give as much as you can afford, for this is your service; your medicine costs "x" shillings.' Then if the patient is very poor but offers a lot, the dispenser refuses; if the patient insists, we use the money to provide him with vitamin-rich food. If the patient is rich but gives little, the dispenser pushes him a bit.

We hope soon to have local committees running each clinic. Ideally, the people of each community should pay some sort of tax to the committee, thus supporting the clinic, building it up if they wish, and eliminating the need for patients to bring money when they come to the doctor. The difficulty is a belief among the mountain people, undoubtedly started by witch-doctors, that the more you pay the better medical service you will receive and thus the healthier you will become when you take your medicines. People won't be satisfied with their treatment unless they pay *at* the clinic when they receive their medicines.

This morning a local teacher came to Masianokeng clinic and told the doctor of a problem he is having difficulty in solving. He explained that a charitable organization of some note has a plan here at two Maseru schools. Every day they supply for all the children who are able to pay a tickee one 'Nutritious biscuit', which is just nutritious enough to be a fair prophylaxis against vitamin deficiency diseases as long as it is taken regularly. Usually only about half the children can afford to pay; those who can't afford the service must go to another part of the room where they sit and watch the richer children (who don't need the programme) line up to receive and eat their biscuits.

The teacher's dilemma is that yesterday, although he had a full, unopened carton of biscuits, only one boy in the class had money. The teacher couldn't decide whether or not he should open the carton just for one child out of the whole class. He's not allowed to give biscuits to those children who can't pay. He told us that he is shocked and upset by the whole plan—for it produces poverty complexes in the children and lacks permanent meaning anyway because once the kids are out of school and not given the biscuit their health depends on, they will starve again. He said, 'My God, you should see the pathetic hunger reflected on the faces of the children who can't afford to pay for these vile-tasting biscuits! It's these, the poorer children, who need the vitamins—and instead of getting them they have to hungrily watch the richer children, who have all the vitamins they need, adding to their full bellies. I'm sure the richer kids wouldn't even eat the things if it weren't that others who can't afford them stand and watch enviously.'

He went on to explain that a further part of the organization's plan is that the children should learn to grow a garden and thus be educated to produce for themselves a more suitable diet. For this purpose, the plan suggests that the children work in a garden to be grown by them at the school. This teacher's school has set up a garden measuring about ten feet by twenty feet for the one hundred and twenty children participating. How does the organization help with the garden? They provide free barbed wire with which the children are to surround the garden for the purpose of keeping animals out. What do the children grow in the garden? Mealies, mealies, and mealies—the starchy food they have been starving on all their lives.

Last night, late in the evening, Carl called on the house phone from the clinic, asking me to come over immediately.

On the examining table was lying a child of about three years of age who was nothing but bones and sagging skin. It hardly looked human. From a bottle suspended above the table, the child was receiving drip feed, and the grandmother, who sat across the room, was staring blankly at the scene. Carl explained to me, somewhat bitterly, that the child has been on the premises for almost a week. A nurse was giving it injections of vitamins every day, and Rosalia was bringing special food for it to eat. This evening the grandmother, who is staying with the child, called the doctor and told him that the baby was having a fit.

I couldn't understand how, if the baby were being taken care of so well, it could now be dying of starvation. Carl explained that the food had been brought as ordered, but that the grandmother had been tossing it away instead of feeding it to the child; when, as in the birth of this baby, the mother dies in childbirth, the grandmother who takes charge of the child will sometimes out of superstition and fear of evil in the child let it die in this way. Also, it is possible that the grandmother believed, as so many people here do, that so long as a patient is getting injections he will automatically be fine. Well, this baby was starving, injections or not. It is disturbing enough that the grandmother never said anything and didn't feed the child the food that was brought, but worse that the highly qualified, registered nurse who gave the baby an injection every day didn't notice that the baby was starving to death, or if she did, said nothing to the doctor. Surely she couldn't help but see the child getting thinner, see its eyes roll uncontrollably in weakness. But she said nothing.

It is impossible to understand such things. And how can we

combat such problems without sufficient staff—staff to educate people and check to see that every patient is being properly taken care of? It is not enough here to provide food; one must see that it is eaten by the patient.

The child died before us.

The BASOMED plane is delayed for another two weeks because the mechanics in the Republic have to send to the States for a new prop. They worked on the plane for a few weeks, fixing the bent wing, and only when ready to return the plane to us did they look to see if they had in stock the correct sized propellor. Needless to say, they hadn't.

Carl and our accountant met with Mr. Betts of OXFAM, and Mr. Betts made some very promising statements. We can now only wait for further developments from him. If only he might realize how much depends on his good will!

I was surprised today to be hailed from across the grounds by a man from Sehlabeng who had travelled from the mountains to Masianokeng to consult Dr. van Aswegen. When I asked after our friends at Sehlabeng, he said, 'They are fine. They have waited a long time for you to return, but they know that you and Molefi haven't deserted them. They know you will both return to work and stay with them.' Molefi and I have been missing Sehlabeng and feeling guilty about our long delay in returning to that village.

I arrived at the Maseru aerodrome yesterday morning, and came to Khubetsoana on a charter plane with the builder, Mr. van Jaarsveld. There are still two more loads of building materials to come up, though all the stuff should have been here long ago. The buildings were made in the Republic to the wrong specifications, weigh over one thousand pounds apiece, and therefore cannot be flown here one per plane-load. This minor error on the part of the company in the Republic is costing us hundreds of pounds and weeks of precious time.

We set right to work at Khubetsoana—very hard work. I'm really not used to such labour, but it feels great to be straining physically instead of mentally. The buildings, steel prefabs, have no plans with them, so getting the parts arranged correctly is a job requiring genius. We have been working on them now for two days, and all five frames are standing. They look great. The work on the site, exhausting as it is, is pleasurable. There's satisfaction in seeing these buildings going up. Also, very, gratifying, there are a few people from the village helping us voluntarily.

The builder, Mr. van Jaarsveld, is friendly, kind and pleasant, if rather taciturn. Most important now, of course, he's a very capable builder—which is, after all, what we hired him for.

We've continued building, though we have been hampered every day by heavy rain. A most frustrating thing is that not all the building parts are drilled correctly, some of them—we have no way of knowing which ones without plans—are still in Maseru at the aerodrome, and no planes can land even when the rains stop for a little while because the clouds are low and the airstrip sopping wet. Tomorrow is Sunday, which means there can be no charter planes coming, and since it appears that it will rain tomorrow, there will be no planes for a few days thereafter. When a plane does finally come, we will have to send a message to the lowlands instructing the doctor to get in touch with the company who constructed the buildings and find out what's going on with these damned parts that don't fit together. It's quite maddening to sit here; we ran out of work today—can do nothing simply because we are out of bolts.

Today while we were putting together the steel frames, climbing all over the roofs, the bells of the Catholic school across the river began to ring out furiously. Looking across the mountains, we could see a man in black dress, a priest, riding towards the building, and swarms of shouting children racing out of the school to meet him. Incited by the school teacher and the mad ringing of the bells, the children were wild with excitement and noise. I asked one of the men working with us, 'What the hell's going on?' He answered with a poker face, "Jesus Christ has arrived.'

It was the priest from Sebesong making a visit—the same priest who had refused to receive the emergency message concerning the doctor's plane accident. I'm sure he was filled with gladness at the sight of our hospital going up for the local people.

A charter plane finally came to Khubetsoana, and we've begun arrangements with the Republic firm about building problems. Not only have we had great trouble with faulty manufacturing of parts, and shortage of parts (a problem which in the isolation of the mountain ranges brings all work to a standstill) but the very design of the buildings seems unsuitable. Because there are no diagonal supports, all chances are that the mountain winds will in not too long a time twist the rectangular shapes into parallelograms.

A charter plane came with Carl and an engineer from the Republic company which constructed the prefabs. We pointed out all the faults, fought for a while with the company representative, and took an unyielding position. An hour later a plane came to pick up Carl and the company man, and now we are again working at trying to get these damned buildings up. It's murder; the extra bolts which were sent up are too long and required five or six washers apiece. Now we're going to run out of washers, and won't be able to go on working until another plane comes. There's no plane scheduled.

On the building site we're working with a few men from the village. It's enjoyable—good, hard and worthwhile work made extra interesting and important by the fact that we are working hand-in-hand with the villagers. It's so frustrating, however, to constantly run into obstacles of missing parts, wrong-sized pieces, and generally faulty design; these buildings should have been up long ago—and now we see that it is only through the ingenuity of our builder, Mr. van Jaarsveld, that there has been any progress at all.

Mr. van Jaarsveld is quite an old man, short and bald, has a grizzly white beard and smokes a plain, big-bowled pipe. His eyes are simple, sometimes sad, and usually kind—but always far from the person whom he's with. He was born in Maseru and has lived all his life in Ladybrand, a small village just across the border in the Republic. Over the years he has constructed what bridges and buildings there are in Basutoland.

We've been living together in this little hut for over two weeks now. He is quiet and unassuming, and eats whatever we have on hand, never complaining. He and I go to bed early, usually with the radio playing classical (he prefers rock and roll, but enjoys passively half-listening to almost any music). At five or six in the morning he makes a pot of thick coffee, Afrikaans style, and wakes me up brightly with, 'Here's some coffee for you, old man.' We have coffee, get up and dressed, make breakfast (sometimes Molopo and Molefi are up in time to eat with us) and then go off to work—usually at about six-thirty. He works with skill and amazing energy, giving everyone incentive by his inexhaustible enthusiasm and momentum. On days when we can't work all day because of thunderstorms and heavy lightning, he becomes depressed—as evidenced by his frustrated restlessness; when we are able to work from early to late without interruption he is elated sometimes to the point of uttering as many as fifty words in the evening.

He seldom speaks or listens except in rare moods. Usually when you address him he answers distractedly, 'Yip, yip, yip.' If you have said something he wants to hear he sort of wakes up, and says, 'Umh, umh, umh,' and blushes with a foolish smile. Then you realize that he is embarrassed at not having listened and repeat for his benefit what you had said. When dinner time comes, I say, 'Well, what will it be? Vienna sausages and mealy meal, or canned beef and mealy meal?' He answers, 'Yip, that's all right, old man.' One night I caught him with, 'How about dill pickles for supper?' The answer, 'Yip, that's all right, old man.'

Limited a companion as he may sound, he's really a perfect person to live with—and he's great on the job, really knows how to work and handle his help. He doesn't get angry at the men who so easily fall into lethargy, but just says, 'Come on Grandpa. If you don't get to work I'll send the "*tokolosi*" after you.' (The *tokolosi* is a spirit feared by the local people; in fact, Moremi at Masianokeng sleeps with cement blocks under the legs of his cot so that the *tokolosi* won't be able to reach him. This is only one of many spirits against which people must protect themselves, including 'the bones', or skeletons, which prowl about at night. The people are full of fears, but I have yet to meet anyone here who is not willing to joke about the spirits.)

We put the roofs on the buildings today. Our hands are all chopped from handling the corrugated-iron edges. The hardest thing is the climbing on slippery and steeply sloped roofs of iron sheeting with the sharp edges being the only things one can hang to to keep from falling. When we begin a roof it is easy to climb around on the rafters, but when we are completing the roof we get stuck on top with steep slopes on each side. However, we have the aid of a rickety ladder made of rotten wooden poles tied together with woven reeds.

The first time I had to come down from a completed roof I was pretty shaky, not being the least bit athletic or in love with heights. My valiant efforts to reach the ground were amusing to everyone but me. I painfully eased myself to a seated position on the two sharp edges of the roof peak, and began to descend by sliding along the roof on my ass while two of the men waited below to grab my feet when I reached the edge. Just as my feet touched the top rung of the ladder and my ankles were grasped by the men below, one guy who was still on the top of the roof ran a wrench along the corrugated-iron ridging, making a sound much like that of a steel building collapsing. The building remained standing, however, while everyone present collapsed—me with terror, the others with sympathetic laughter.

I got rather fed up today with the slow progress of the work on the airstrip and also with the difficulty we are having getting horses for travel. On the airstrip, in order to level the ground, much dirt has to be brought from a distant area and placed into craters on the strip. As we have nothing with which to move the dirt, the men have been attempting to carry huge hunks of sod on their heads. It is painfully slow and difficult work. All our efforts to locate a sledge and oxen have failed; one man nearby owns a a sledge, but refuses to let us use it for less than ten shillings a day—a high price here. Secondly, with the problem of availability of horses, we are also running into lack of help from the people. It is necessary for Molefi and me to ride to and from Mantsonyane (a day each way) to see the trader there about his helping us set up a drug depot near his store. Now we find that the local people refuse to let us borrow horses, and we have no way of travelling.

Though the people here are as anxious to have a hospital as are the people at nearby places such as Mohokare and Likhoiting, they have become complacent because they see us building and have had the doctor's services for some time without any great effort on their part. The people at villages where we have not begun even the first steps of a medical service are contributing funds, working on airstrips for no fee, lending huts and horses gladly and immediately, and building clinic buildings themselves. Here they gave us a large and beautiful piece of land with two fountains, gave us temporarily their own homes as shelter, and a few people are helping build for no payment—but the local chiefs, with the exception of Chief Thaba of this village, have done little, and the majority of the people feel that the hospital will go up and the service survive and grow whether they help out or not. They're wrong.

We must meet with the local chiefs to remind them that this hospital will be only so big as they wish it to be, and that what it will provide for their people depends on them. We expect to have at least voluntary help for the building of the airstrip and huts, as well as horses available to us whenever we require them for work which furthers the effectiveness of the clinic. If they will not go so far as to do this little bit right now for themselves, we will simply pour our greatest efforts into some other village where the people give more material evidence of wanting a hospital.

Tsamai, our local friend, has given me some insight into the reason for the local people's unwillingness to enthusiastically help themselves. He explained that despite our efforts to make clear our financial situation, most of the people think that BASOMED is the richest organization in Basutoland (for, after all, we have a plane, wear comparatively rich clothing, and can afford to occasionally eat meat). It is also everyone's impression that the government is giving us unlimited amounts of money, and that they gave us the aeroplane—the fact being, of course, that the government has given us only antagonism and not a cent of aid.

As Molefi and I were walking back from the building site the other evening, we saw a bunch of kids crowded around a man who was sitting on the ground concentrating intensely on something. I asked Molefi what was going on, and he answered matter-of-factly, 'That's a plumber; you don't see them too often in the mountains.'

We went over for a closer look, and found this man sitting with a metal wash-basin in his lap, working on it with a few crude tools; around him on the ground were a few more beaten-up basins. He had a large tin can from which he took a small piece of tin. Placing the scrap of metal in a hole in the basin, he pounded it with something like a hammer into the consistency of solder, thus, after extreme effort, patching the hole quite effectively. All the people of the village who are rich enough to have basins, usually old ones which are full of holes and generally falling apart, bring them to this man for repair whenever he visits. He works with fixed attention, repairing things with remarkable care where often we couldn't discover what was to be fixed. I never saw such initiative in the Sehlabeng area—but, then again, I never saw basins there.

We've been living well for the past two days. We bought a sheep which is delicious and every night we have a roast; we cook sometimes on a kerosene stove, and when we run out of fuel we use 'Basuto coal'—horse manure dried and bricked. There is a woman in the village, a lovely person, who insists on bringing us '*shishe monate*' every morning. It is a thin porridge made slightly sour by fermentation of the mealies which make it up—very good. Also, as it is now the height of the mealy season, we are constantly getting gifts of fresh maize; at the site in the afternoon people bring some to us, and in the evenings the woman who is lending us her hut brings in armfuls of the cobs. Much better than the dried and crushed mealies we eat all year as mealy meal.

We are almost through with the buildings, and they look beautiful —a dream come true. Many people are coming to the site now, marvelling at this new kind of building they see. A few old women are helping us carry water for cement, in huge three-gallon cans on their heads; they carry them with the water about half an inch from the top, and the can is so heavy that I can hardly lift it; across fields and over mountains they carry it without spilling a drop and without showing any exhaustion. There is one young woman hanging around all the time who has a loud, merry voice and a steady smile which easily becomes a laugh. She brightens our days.

Today while we worked about thirty children came and sang songs for us, dancing and clapping as they sang and casting shy but attention-seeking glances at us. There is nothing so exhilarating and warming as watching these children, ranging in age from three to fifteen, singing or just running about.

The building is hard work—sweating under the hot sun for

nine hours without break but for an occasional swallow of coffee or Basuto beer. The men from the village who are working with us are a fine bunch, really tops, and much kidding accompanies the work. Today, for example, one man got an ant in his shoe—one of the ants so numerous here, about an inch long and with ferocious jaws.

He hopped about for a long time before finally crushing the menace, and now he is working extra hard since we pointed out to him that he shouldn't have been standing still on the job. He insists that Mr. van Jaarsveld finally set the *tokolosi* on him as he is always threatening to do. He, incidentally, is the same man, who, after teasing me about my dislike for roof work, was afraid to go to the top of the buildings when we asked him to. Now he is happy to stay on the roofs, where there are no ants.

One of the men is an old character who looks like a retired boxer. He is of large build with heavy hanging features, talks in a dull whine, and always wears a heavy overcoat (which is in shreds) despite the intense sun. He is in fact no dope, but seems at first extremely dull and sluggish because he sleeps on his feet like a horse. We must constantly prod him to wakefulness, but are glad to have his help because he is such a well-meaning guy. It's impossible to stop his dozing off on the job; I ask him from the roof of a building to hand me a bucket of water, and he starts from his sleep and goes to get a hammer. Today we all nicknamed him 'Grandma' and he is feeling pretty grouchy about it. When we call him by the name he refuses to answer, and when pushed a bit he whines and mumbles in resentment, before finally laughing heartily with everyone else.

The thing I'm constantly being kidded about is my American accent in speaking Sesotho—an accent never before heard here. Everyone waits for me to open my mouth and let loose with this strange dialect. They laugh a lot about it, but are conducting a massive effort to help me improve; they glow whenever I utter a word they thought I hadn't known.

This evening, Montere, our apprentice dispenser and a very capable school teacher, was taking shelter in our hut from a violent hail storm. Suddenly, as we sat talking and smoking our green Basuto tobacco, he pointed excitedly out of the door and exclaimed, 'Yes, he's changed the hail to rain!' Startled by these strange words, I exclaimed, 'What?' Montere repeated his words, and explained that there is a witch-doctor in the village who keeps away hail. He lives at the chief's residence and is paid in crops by all the villagers to keep away ice storms.

Molefi, after he had stopped laughing at my disbelief, pointed out to me that once when he had washed some clothes at the river and had left them on the bank to dry, he had been ordered by the chief to move them immediately or face arrest; the witch-doctor won't allow clothes to be dried at the river because it causes hail. Also, once while we were working at the site we were visited by a representative of the chief who ordered us to stop breaking stones at midday. It hadn't meant anything to me at the time, but now Molefi explained that breaking stones at midday causes hail.

Montere told me excitedly of another power this witch-doctor has: he can make lightning strike anywhere, and anyone, he wishes. He flies up in the air, hovers over his victim, and strikes him with lightning. He failed only once, Montere says, and as he later explained to the villagers in apology, 'When I flew up to the sky and took my position above him, I saw that he was sitting on the ground holding a sword up in the air. If I threw lightning on him, I would definitely have fallen and landed on the sword. I flew some distance away, and then returned later only to find that he was still holding up the weapon, so I had to spare him in order to avoid my own death.'

Because I doubted the validity of this story, Montere insists on introducing me to this man, and dares me to sit in a hut while the witch-doctor throws lightning at me.

When I questioned Montere's rational sense in believing in such magic, he told me that he had learned in school that 'No one really knows what causes lightning.'

Later I said to Molefi, 'How can a person like Montere, a school-teacher, believe in such things?' He answered with a bit of confusion, 'Yes, surely these things aren't true—are they?' I said, 'Well, damned if I'm going to sit in a hut while some witch-doctor throws lightning at me in order to find out!' We laughed away the problem gratefully.

I find myself these nights looking forward to the moon's coming up just as I used to look forward to a good play or concert in

New York. Really, it is a thrill to see it come up over the mountains, covering the ragged land with a hard blue light. Except for its chilly bluish tint, it's almost like sunlight in brightness; as the moon rises, the edges of the light it casts are sharply defined and creep up slowly on the shadows, scattering them into the valleys.

We decided two days ago to call community meetings, or *pitsos*, at Mohokare and this village, Khubetsoana. Tsamai and the chief agreed to lend us horses.

Tsamai took our clinic budget and offered to translate it into Sesotho for the few people who can read. It is valuable for presentation at the *pitsos*, so he did the huge job. On the bottom of the sheet where we had written, 'This plan is devised to help you help yourselves—please co-operate,' Tsamai added, 'WAKE UP AND HELP YOURSELVES.'

The *pitsos*, however, turned out to be most disappointing. Each of the villages in the area has its own local chief, and above all the chiefs is the area chief, Morena Mohokare, who is also chief of the village of Ha Mohokare. Therefore, our meetings had to be organized through Chief Mohokare, and unfortunately he is not reliable. When we arrived at his village after two hours of riding, we found that no one had been notified of the *pitso* and we ended up addressing about thirty people while there should have been hundreds if word had been properly spread by the chief.

The *pitso* at Ha Mohokare, small as it was, served to bring out the great and obvious difficulty that faces us: the people here are so used to having what there is *given* to them, and are so accustomed to being exploited when things are sold to them, that they can hardly understand the concept of self-help. We try to explain and then say that we need their help for themselves in putting up a hospital and levelling an airstrip; the reaction, except from the most perceptive, is, 'Do you expect us to work and then pay for medical treatment as well?' After about two hours of explanation and discussion at Ha Mohokare, however, they came round, due largely to efforts on the part of those who did understand to make the others catch on. By the time we had finished, with a firm, 'Come on and get moving if you ever want to live healthily!' they offered support and even became enthusiastic. People wanted to contribute money, but I didn't feel sure that the project was fully understood, and couldn't bring myself to accept the idea of contributions just now. Besides, they might think that by giving a bit of money their obligations would be finished and they themselves entitled to free medical service and medicines (they don't comprehend that we have to pay for the medicines we give them). I asked them instead of giving money to come and pitch into the work on the site, and some men volunteered to come on Monday. Of course by Monday much of the enthusiasm of the moment might have died, but if they want a hospital enough they'll give their help Monday or the next day.

A few remarks to show their typical conditioning: I told them that BASOMED has no money as they believe it has, but that the money for these five buildings we have put up came from a foundation in London who agreed to help them help themselves. I said that now the money is used up and it is for them to work from this bare start. In response to this reasoning, one man asked, 'Why don't you ask the organization in England for more money?' He wasn't being sarcastic, he just thought that people who care should give whatever is needed. I told him that even if we had another million pounds, we would not give it to them because we know that if they really want a hospital they will use the beginning we have given them to make a really fine hospital for themselves.

I spoke very strongly to them, and afterwards Tsamai backed up my speech with a really fiery one. It was a huge effort to force understanding upon them; they many times expressed their anxiety to have a hospital, but could not comprehend that we were treating them as adults, and not trying to exploit them as fools.

It wasn't too bad, but really took all our energy—and surely there remain many misconceptions. I think it will all work out well with time, and when they see from our actions that we mean what we say.

Next we rode back to Khubetsoana to see Chief Thaba and hold the second *pitso*. We found the situation there, no one knowing of the *pitso*, to be the same as at Ha Mohokare. We had a good long talk with the chief, however, at his home. He's an impressive guy, understands fully, as he showed clearly by a number of comments, and trusts that we are sincere. He has made numerous efforts to help us, for example, giving us horses, donkeys, sledge and oxen at the site. And he has run into the same problems that we have apparently—people insisting, 'You should pay high wages for work.'

Chief Thaba is sure that once the hospital is running and a committee is formed, people will catch on. He says that the two hundred pounds estimated cost per month for running a hospital is not beyond the capabilities of the thousands of people in the area, and that when they see the hospital working and have their own committee to help them understand, it will come easily.

As we took leave of Chief Thaba, he said to us, 'We won't give up! We'll keep trying again and again until we succeed. Meeting such a man snapped me out of my feeling of intense discouragement, but my anger increases every moment when I think that in the guise of altruism men will remove the backbones from a nation's people through giving to them without teaching them.

Tomorrow morning, if the weather holds, we go off to Masianokeng by Lockheed. I need the change of pace, and to see Carl, very much.

February 21 —March 29, 1963

Monday morning at Khubetsoana we were up at sunrise, packed and ready for the plane. A plane came sure enough, but buzzed low over the airstrip and went off, not returning. Not having seen a note drop, we couldn't figure out why the pilot had made one pass and gone away. We searched the airstrip and surrounding cornfields for an hour hoping to find a note, but no such luck.

It was maddening not knowing what was happening and not being able to go anywhere far from the strip for fear that the plane would come back in our absence. For two days we waited for an aeroplane, running out of precious cigarettes the first day and smoking green Basuto tobacco which we rolled in any paper we could find lying around the hut. With tired heads and sore throats, we waited endlessly for the sound of a plane coming our way, jumping up and running to the airstrip for numerous false alarms, sound mirages caused by the mountain winds.

A pilot finally flew in with a Lockheed, telling us that he had dropped an explanatory note two days ago in a nearby mealie field. He was quite surprised when we said we hadn't found it.

I arrived back at Masianokeng to find that the doctor had finally, thank goodness, taken a much-needed rest for a week or two. He had been ready to collapse, mentally and physically. He has left me in charge, and I'm struggling along, trying not only to keep things going but to put things in order: correspondence, personal staff problems, transport of building materials to various mountain areas, and the building of a drug depot here with Mr. van Jaarsveld. So far all is going as smoothly as can be expected.

As anxious as I am to see Carl, I'm much relieved that he

finally made the right decision on this need for a rest. His plane isn't available anyway, so this is an opportune time for him to leave. It's the first vacation he's had since he started this work six years ago.

It was wonderful to return home. When I walked in, young Thabiso, the Christmas-adopted son, cried out and ran over to me, throwing his arms around me and saying over and over again, 'I'm so happy to see you, *Ntati* Jeff.' Later when I went to speak with him for a while, he kept on beaming and saying over and over again, '*Kanete, ke thabile haholo,*' 'Really, I am so happy.' He is doing me the honour in Carl's absence of sleeping on the couch in my room, and I learn by the minute and feel intensely warmed as I sit writing in the evenings to the sound of his steady breathing. He sleeps with a smile on his face and just seems to be a bundle of all that is good and innocent. He's a devil, of course, but that's why we love him.

Rosalia came in and hugged me until I was blue and gasping for air. She kissed me and held my head in her hands, finally putting her head on my shoulder and just swallowing me into her huge motherly body. She has been preparing gourmet dinners from nothing since I came, and is determined to stuff me even if she has to shovel the food into my mouth.

I found in the post a letter we have been waiting months for: a personal letter to Carl from Dr. Schweitzer saying that he hopes his friends all over the world will give their support to Carl's work. Apart from the obvious fund-raising value of this letter, it has a meaning to Carl beyond expression. Dr. Schweitzer's philosophy and work, which are inseparable, have been a profound inspiration to him.

Masianokeng,
P.O. Box 169,
Maseru,
Basutoland.

Dear Colleague,

Pardon me that I write only now. I had so much work that I could not keep my correspondence the way I wished. A thousand thanks for your dear letter, in which you reported about your work. You know, of course, what regard I have for your work ('Werk') and its success. I know what difficulties you have to gather the means for the establishment of your hospital. But I hope that my friends in the world offer you their interest and help you with gifts for your hospital, which has so great a significance for the area in which you are active. How I would like to come to you to become better acquainted with your work, but I am tied down by my work at Lambarene.

With best thoughts I am devotedly yours

Albert Schweitzer.

Lambaréné
9 Februar 1963

In the afternoon we were visited by the school-teacher, Cardwell Mciteka, who just wanted to see that everything was OK and to offer his services for anything which might come along. I like this man, one of the BASOMED committee members, more every time I see him, and I see him quite often. He is sincere, kind, friendly and a man of action as well as a man who is fearless towards adverse opinion. Some of the other committee members would do well to learn from him.

My favourite of the patients at Masianokeng, a middle-aged woman whom we call simply 'Mama', complained to me of intense pains when I first went over to see her at the clinic. She is suffering from tuberculosis of the hip, and recovering well now. I have been visiting her regularly since my return, and now she is beaming all the time and telling me that she feels wonderful and must be all better. She gets around on crutches, and has such a perfect disposition that she has become part of the family here. Her daughter, Margaret, is also a joy to have around; she is about seven and is always twisted up with shyness. I give her sweets every day, but when I speak with her she just puts her hands behind her back, twists around sideways, giggles, and sticks her tongue out of the side of her mouth . . . all the while watching me coyly. Beautiful child, and always as happy as she can possibly be.

Bethuel is at Morija Hospital, the Protestant Mission Hospital quite some distance from here, recovering from his tuberculosis. He is being well taken care of at Morija, and though immobilized by a cast, is able to get schooling at the hospital. He went calmly, with resignation and hope—qualities in which people here excel. I must somehow get there to visit him.

Mr. van Jaarsveld came this morning to Masianokeng to begin arrangements for the building of the drug depot being put on our premises by a South African drug company. It is a twelve by forty-eight foot building. The company will pay for everything, including the builder's wages, and will supply us with medical stock for distribution to our clinics, at, of course, discount prices.

Mr. van Jaarsveld and I have become strangely good friends. He is very sympathetic to our work, and gives us all the free help he can. Monday he is moving in with us here until the depot is finished, and this morning he brought us as a gift from his small farm in Ladybrand some fresh sausage and a bottle of wine brandy, which tastes like home brew and may very well be.

Rosalia tells me every time she sees me that I mustn't shave off my beard (which I allowed to grow while in the mountains). Every time we pass each other she stops, and strokes my cheek, saying, 'It's so nice. You mustn't shave it, Jeff—please don't take it off. It's so nice!' I'm anxious to shave off the damn thing; the only reason I grew the itching bush was that I had no razor in the mountains. This morning, however, I was caught just before the act by Rosalia who came running into the washroom with a local woman and said, 'Stop! Stop! She told me yesterday that she likes your beard very much and that you really mustn't shave it off. Please leave it, Jeff. It's so nice.' She clasped her hands before her and swooned, then hurried off.

Upon sneaking back to the washroom later to shave off the beard despite all protests, I found every razor had disappeared.

A girl from the Republic came to visit us yesterday, but left hurriedly after one brief encounter with Basuto custom. She was walking down the hill to the shop when suddenly stones started sailing past her, a few of them narrowly missing her head. She whirled about, and saw a man across the road lobbing the rocks from behind a bush. She ran on in a panic, and the man followed her all the way to the shop, continuing to bombard her dangerously.

By local custom, when a man sees a woman with whom he wishes to sleep he hurls stones at her; if she doesn't want his affections, she picks up one of his stones and throws it on past her—at which point he graciously leaves her alone. Our pretty visitor, not knowing the proper thing to do, accepted his proposal and teased him by running away.

The huge amount of work that has piled up here, and the confusion of keeping the operation together, is driving me nuts. Exhaustion and, worse, frustration.

The other evening Nurse Mini arrived by charter plane from the mountains, bringing with her a patient who was in agony. He had a disease of the bladder which made him totally unable to urinate, and though he bore his pain without complaint, he was obviously suffering terribly. We persuaded Joe Mapetla to drive him to Maseru hospital in his Mercedes.

As we walked down the corridors of the hospital, and then through the surgical ward, I wondered how this man was reacting inwardly to this entirely strange world where he was to be handled by just as strange people. He appeared dazed and horrified by the too sudden appearance of something so new to him as we led him slowly along. I wished he could have been treated in surroundings more familiar to him for surely his pain was enough without the shock and fright of exposure to a modern hospital after a life in mud huts.

It's a good thing Mini returned to Masianokeng, for I don't know what would have been the result of this morning's trauma had she not been here. It was about four in the morning when Boitjke, the doctor's Alsatian who sleeps by my bed in the doctor's absence, started whining annoyingly. I figured that he was just pitying himself for being without Carl for so long, but unable to sleep for the noise, I got out of bed, grabbed him by the scruff of the neck, and dragged him outside, slamming the door behind him. I lay in bed then for about an hour, still unable to sleep—feeling rotten about having treated the animal so nastily; also for some reason I felt slightly ill at ease, partly because Thabiso was awake on the couch across the room and radiating uneasiness. Suddenly Josepha came running into the room, and told me to come quickly because Rosalia was ill.

I ran half-dressed out to her rondavel to find her gasping futilely for breath and shaking in frightening spasms. Nurse Mini, however, was there and knew just what to do. Rosalia suffers from serious asthma and this morning was having a bad attack. Mini treated her and I held Rosalia's head for an hour before we managed to get hold of someone with a car to take her to the hospital in Maseru. She regained full consciousness late in the morning at the hospital, and this evening her condition is much improved.

They treated her with encouraging kindness at the hospital.

Mr. van Jaarsveld has been staying with us at Masianokeng for a while now. His little-old-builder characteristics stand out much more prominently here than in the mountains. He never seats himself in a position for conversation, but always places himself in a dark corner of the room when everyone else is congregated in the centre. You walk through the centre-room, and suddenly become aware of his presence. There he sits, hour upon hour, in a dark corner of the room never saying a word. When a guest comes in to visit, I force Mr. van Jaarsveld to come into a seat in the centre of the room and have a drink with us. He sits there without a word, despite our efforts to bring him into the conversation. His silence allows guests to make statements starting with, 'Just between you and me . . .' in forgetfulness of the builder's presence. Then, suddenly, in the middle of a conversation, he comes to life with, 'Jeff, old man, I don't think that beam is going to fit.'

Mr. van Jaarsvald shows me everything he does. I'll be sitting at the desk in the house struggling with massive piles of correspondence when Thabiso comes in and tells me that the builder is calling me ('*Mohaha ua bitsa, n'tati*'). I desert my work, go outside to the site of the depot, and ask Mr. van Jaarsveld what he wants. 'You see, old man, I'm one-fourth inch short on the foundation this end, and can't understand as it's all square.' After this comes a long explanation accompanied by lengthy measurements to prove that the difficulty exists. I suppress the rising, 'Hell, you're the expert, man . . . I don't understand what you're talking about.' Instead I nod my head sympathetically, and say, 'Well, does it matter much?' 'No, I can fix it easily, old man,' he answers. 'Good show, man, carry on,' I say, and return to my desk and try to pull together my frayed mind.

He really is an easy person to have around—though I'll never figure out why I enjoy his company so much.

On Friday morning I had to hitch-hike to the village of Mantsonyane at the end of the mountain road to arrange for our use of a drug depot there and to find people willing to provide weekly donkey transport of supplies from Mantsonyane to our various mountain clinics.

While there I visited the unfinished Anglican mission hospital, where an administrator said to me, 'I can't understand why BASOMED is non-denominational. What on earth is the value of your work if it is non-denominational?' And later, 'Of course we take any patient in, but we much prefer to use our scanty accommodation for those who are heathens and can be converted.' I wondered, is he running a hospital or what? Could it be that the Catholic missions hold a similar view, that they're so intent on the religious angle that the medical matters don't count to them? Perhaps they figure that our service isn't worth anything since it converts no one.

I'm reminded of a story Carl tells me of a local priest, once his close friend, who one day claimed that he had figured out what is the biggest trouble in this country—the reason for the people being starved and diseased. He said, 'One day I looked out over my school classes, and saw all these emaciated boys and girls. I said to myself, "I bet all these boys and girls are masturbating! Why else would they all be so sickly?"' The Father explained how he had sent all the girls out of the room, and after telling the boys to cover their eyes, had asked all those who masturbated to raise their hands. He exclaimed, 'Every one of those boys but two raised his hand! No wonder the people of this country are so poor and sick.' The doctor told the Father what he thought of his theories, and said, 'Surely, Father, you must have masturbated at some time in your life.' The Father replied angrily 'My sex life is none of your business.'

What a relief it was to return to Masianokeng and to the wonderful people with whom I find happiness. As I walked from the road towards the house, Thabiso and Sechlobi came running out and shook my hands; Moremi came and dragged me to his hut to try his new motor bike, and Nurse Mini and I spent the afternoon together.

Another dispenser soon came to join us, and showed me a letter he had written in English to a girl he had met on a train. I was so delighted with the letter that he gave me permission to make copies of it. Such poetry. . .

Dear Eleanor,

One day there will be a sigh, and what had been life dumb would become a simple joy. I thought faithful, close to receive your letter on Monday the 25th of this month waiting for my arrival. I even thought of that simple silence we met in that enjoyable compartment we were. I thought you of a centre from which my life can radiate into its ways. Far as you are but you was my earth. My roots of love were in you, dark and close and strong, and what flowered in you depended on 'LOVE'.

You made it a surprise. It was only on Monday the 25th of February when I come in my room and find you (your letter) waiting for me. Actually waiting for my attention. I never thought that you will do it. Trust me or not, it is true; praise cannot deceive when one has in him/herself the feel of her/his own hands; the knowledge of what is good. Believe it love is so. Consider how plain and natural it is my dear, that it should be so. Do you not appreciate sharing it with me?

Your letter came over my memory like sweet sound that breathes upon a bank of violets (flowers), stealing and giving odour. The unseen force is drawing me fast to itself. For the love of heavens, of justice, of generosity, of the honour of your name I wait for your favourable reply.

If I profane you with my unwealthiest words this holy shrine, the gentle sin is that my apologies are ready stand to smooth that rough touch with a tender humbleness.

With best wishes of love I end,

Your,

ALFRED MOLOPO

Last night at nine o'clock I was sitting in the lounge having coffee when behind me I heard Carl's voice say, 'Well hello.' I jumped about five feet—couldn't believe he was finally home. He and I went into his room and talked for an hour; he thanked me profusely for everything, said that every morning he felt like calling on the phone to thank me for taking over for him.

When it was time for him to make the rounds and see everyone, I told him once more how wonderful it was to see him again and have him back. He answered, 'Well, I'm in charge now, so if anyone gets upset you can tell me about it and then fix up the situation yourself.'

While Carl and I were speaking, Thabiso came in. He bowed and clapped his hands a few times as is the custom of loving and respectful greeting, and then threw his arms around Carl.

The whole house changed immediately with his arrival. Everyone was suddenly elated, unable to sleep though it was the middle of the night. This morning there are about fifty patients waiting to see him—and none of us knows how they knew Carl was back.

Our days have been full. Patients are pouring in to see the doctor and we have to prepare all eight mountain clinics for the commencement of the new programme (get nurses to each, organize committees for each clinic, establish embryos of social plans, and so on). The burden of administrative problems, especially that of solving the debt, keeps us more than ever before from the only truly important thing: the work itself for the patients.

It didn't take one day after Carl's return for him to begin feeling the old strains, as evidenced by a subtle undertone of despair and exhaustion in his voice. He never, however, loses his power to act effectively and inspire those around him to do the same.

Three days ago, early in the morning, we received a call from the aerodrome in Maseru informing us that our plane had arrived repaired from the Republic. We didn't do anything about it all morning, but just avoided the topic. At four in the afternoon, Carl came in and said in a voice attempting to be careless, but quaking a bit nevertheless, 'I'm going to Maseru to pick up the plane. Wouldn't you like to come along?' He looked rather pale, and it was almost as if I could see his nerves drawn tight under his skin; hearing his words I soon arrived at an identical condition. This is a psychological battle we both have to win, however, if we are to go on with this work.

We got a quick lift into Maseru aerodrome, and found the plane waiting—crouched as if about to pounce viciously upon us. As though it weren't bad enough to have to fly in it again, we also had to face the matter of testing out a new type of tyre. The small ones are replaced by huge balloon tyres which theoretically are ideal for our type of flying; finding out the truth of their reliability, however, was no game. We felt like test pilots climbing into an X-15.

Carl revved her up, minutely checked all the controls, and taxied slowly to the beginning of the long airstrip. He went over the controls once again, and then taxied back to the hangar. A few checks on the innards of the plane, and then back to the strip again. Off we went, in the oddest manner. We went down the strip, bouncing around like a rubber ball on our new wheels, helpless as we bounded up and down, never touching ground long enough to pick up airspeed. Finally, in one desperate leap, we found the air and stayed up. Then, shaky as hell, testing the plane's every function in the air, we flew to Masianokeng, took a look at the little strip, and flew back to Maseru to practise landing and taking off a few times.

After a few runs, up, down, and up at Maseru, Carl felt he had mastered it. The flabby wheels make landing distance much shorter and more comfortable, but on take-off there is little steering control and a tendency to bounce up and down helplessly. However, with a super effort to hold the nose to the ground until we had reached full air speed, Carl was able to control the bouncing almost completely. We flew to Masianokeng, arriving at sunset, and holding our breath the while landed perfectly despite a hazardous cross wind. Phew! We ran into the house and hit the brandy bottle.

Despite our having lost all our guts for flying, we had to go to Mafisa the next morning. It was a tough flight, and we both felt quite nauseated with uneasiness as we took off from Masianokeng. By the end of the terrifying day, however, we had made the rounds of the mountains, north and south, and had survived it.

People are ecstatic to see the plane back; we couldn't land in many places because of heavy winds across the strips, but as we buzzed over clinic villages people waved and shouted (thinking we can hear them as if we were riding by on horseback). As anxious as we were to land at Sehlabeng, a landing long overdue, it was impossible—but as we came over the village, hundreds of people came streaming out of their huts and flowed in a mass towards the airstrip. A remarkable, and saddening sight. We only hope we'll be able to land there next week.

Flying over the mountains in a Super Cub is a strange sensation. While the stable Cub is known to be the safest plane for such conditions, one feels ever so much more secure in a larger plane. The reasons are, perhaps, that in a larger plane when you look around you see something solid carrying you rather than flimsy canvas; you have the comfort in a larger plane of having someone sitting beside you, while in a small plane there is nothing beside you but void, the passenger and pilot sitting one behind the other; and in the larger plane the motor sounds powerful, not like a motorbike engine.

I find a rare communication in flying with Carl in the Cub. I've picked up some knowledge of what is going on (and wish for my comfort I hadn't), but even with my eyes closed I can feel when he is tense over something. Discussing the day's flying with him, I can spot every moment of the flight which had held danger, judging just from having felt Carl's moods. Flying together, especially in this battle against fear left by the accident, we become closer than brothers. If friendship is based on trust, then this is the height of friendship—for I put myself completely in Carl's hands whenever I step into that plane.

We have been totally unable to relax. Even if in the evenings we manage to get rid of the hordes of visitors frequenting this place like a hotel, quiet talks don't do much to alleviate our problems. Last night Carl and I decided to get away from here for a bit, and so went into town; we needed the day's mail anyway and were out of both brandy and cigarettes.

We drove into town with Mr. van Jaarsveld, in his truck, and headed for the pub. There we met some old friends and had a few drinks. By the time we left at eleven or twelve, Carl was high and I was numb; my teeth felt novocained. It was just what we needed—a change of scene and a diversion from difficulties which are plaguing us constantly. We were laughing all evening, couldn't stop smiling. How rare it was!

To add to the evening's pleasure, we received an encouraging piece of news. The top director of OXFAM is going to be in

Maseru Tuesday on a visit, and Mr. Betts, the local OXFAM representative, has called an important meeting of the BASOMED executive for Sunday 'in preparation for some good news' (as he told Joe Mapetla).

Also it appears that we may finally have found a competent administrative couple—old friends of Carl's who are fascinated by the position and who have excellent qualifications. They will be coming soon to see us.

Two days ago our good friend and executive committee member, Cardwell Mciteka, came to visit. He's as frank and bright a person as one can hope to meet anywhere—a real anomaly here in the lowlands of Basutoland. He and I sat talking for quite a while; he was anxious to ask me numerous questions about the coming meeting with Mr. Betts—for purposes unknown to me. Then Carl came in, and the routine was repeated until Cardwell was satisfied that we knew nothing about whatever he was preparing to tell us.

We urged him to tell us what was on his mind, but he was hesitant because he felt that Joe Mapetla, the chairman of the committee, should have said something to us, and didn't want to do anything behind Joe's back. However, he did feel compelled to speak openly about the matter, which was apparently upsetting him greatly.

Finally he explained that OXFAM, through Mr. Betts, has issued a report which Joe should have brought us by this time. It seems from this report, and from talk Cardwell has heard, that Carl is about to get shafted. Apparently OXFAM is working in conjunction with the local government in giving us a loan: OXFAM to pay two-thirds of our nine thousand pound debt and the government to give us a subsidy of two shillings per patient (each patient costs us approximately twelve shillings).

There are certain conditions to these monies: the doctor being 'too unpractical' for this sort of work, we must find an administrator immediately and the doctor must be deprived of all administrative responsibility. In other words, the doctor would no longer be director of BASOMED, nor would he even be on the executive committee, but would be present at meetings only as 'medical advisor'.

The executive committee must be changed to a managing

committee consisting of three people, one of whom must be a government appointee, and there must be an executive subcommittee also with a government man represented. I can't help noting at this point that the government regularly gives much more substantial subsidies to mission hospitals throughout the country without such inteference stipulations.

The administrator is to be paid by OXFAM a yearly salary of fifteen hundred pounds, thus making him directly responsible to them, not to BASOMED; the doctor would be paid a salary of eighteen hundred pounds per year with which he might do whatever he likes. The doctor's salary would be taken from donation money only—from patients and outside contributors.

No action at all could be taken without the affirmation of the managing committee, and no progressive steps could be taken with new grants until the doctor's debts were paid in full. No grants could be accepted without OXFAM's approval, and once found acceptable by them would be paid towards a solution of the debt, even if there were other needs involved as pressing as the survival of a patient.

And the greatest catch of all: in return for their loan OXFAM demands a full bond on the BASOMED property, and the right to close that bond should they be dissatisfied with the shape of things one year from the date of the loan.

Cardwell's report upset us. At one time, by Carl's own initiative, in his efforts to make the executive committee become more active on its own, he resigned as chairman of that committee. But now his removal from all BASOMED policy-making is being proposed.

We fear that with a government-controlled administration nothing would get done. Politics and the realities of human suffering are virtually unrelated; statistics do not speak the language of human lives and values. We have seen government-run services in operation; they contain nothing of Carl's feeling for the people our work serves, nothing of his dedication and sensitivity to their health and happiness. BASOMED is meaningful to the one hundred thousand people in the mountains as other services aren't because Carl has insisted on the patients coming first.

Were Carl to be removed from the running of BASOMED (and he is just humble enough to let it happen without strong enough protest), and were BASOMED to become like other government services, all would be lost to these mountain people. Cardwell is so upset by this possibility that he vows he will quit should the OXFAM offer be accepted.

In our present difficulties it appears that we have little choice but to accept the OXFAM offer, or watch Carl go bankrupt and the service immediately dissolve. A last-ditch fund-raising effort promises little hope. We are surprised that Betts (and Dr. Clark of the government, who is evidently concerned in this) has suggested these terms to us, knowing the nature of our service and our fear of seeing it reduced to a statistical cypher. The whole thing worries us: OXFAM's plan to make the administrator directly responsible to them rather than to BASOMED; OXFAM's apparent link with the government; the removal of Carl's influence in one quick stroke; and—the Damocles sword above it all—the full bond on our property with the right to close 'if dissatisfied after one year', a vague criterion at best.

But above all we wonder, how close is the connection between OXFAM and the British government?

On Sunday afternoon the meeting with Mr. Betts took place. The committee convened in the apartment of Mrs. Nicholas, the owner of Maseru's hotel, member of the committee, and good friend of Mr. Betts. We were a nervous bunch as we sat in our finest dress, waiting in hushed silence for the arrival of Mr. Betts.

Finally he entered—dressed in tennis shorts and a T-shirt. Despite his informality, however, the meeting took place in an atmosphere of tension, and clarified little. Carl opened with half-hearted thanks to Mr. Betts, and said that Betts's memorandum (which had turned out to be quite a battery against himself) was quite interesting. Everyone mumbled courteous agreement, and no one added anything. Mr. Betts realized that his memo was considered by all to be a presumption, if not much worse, and found himself being rather apologetic to a group of statues, saying, 'Look, now, I'm not trying to tell you how to run things, I'm not trying to hold a pistol to your heads—but surely you see my position. Really, I apologize if I've insulted anyone, but . . . OK, I admit, I am holding a pistol to your heads, but I had no choice but to do so.' It turns out that he has spoken with our creditors already, explaining that he is making an offer which will cover our debts. It would hardly do for us to refuse now, would it, with our creditors waiting for an indication of our good faith?

Cardwell was the first to blurt out his anger, all futile now, after the fact. He added, 'I don't trust the government, I'm suspicious of the motives behind this subsidy offer.' Betts smoothly assured us that he had no intention of putting us at the mercy of the government and was sure that Dr. Clark wouldn't think of doing such a thing.

The meeting flared up briefly again when Carl defended himself against some of the statements in the memorandum. For example, Mr. Betts had said that the doctor had the bad habit of doing things without consulting his committee, when the fact is that the committee members seldom get up a quorum when called together, and know nothing about what is going on in the mountains despite our efforts to explain. Busy as we are, we cannot constantly be travelling into Maseru for abortive meetings. Yet as much as possible we have tried going out of our way to consult the members on every major action.

Throughout the proceedings I struggled to keep my mouth shut, and sat waiting breathlessly for Carl to lose control and blurt out, 'This offer is unacceptable to us.' He was kept from saying it, however, by the immediate threat of our services ending through bankruptcy, through our creditors' prior knowledge of Mr. Betts's proposal, and by the strong possibility that any refusal of OXFAM's deal would have permanent, destructive consequences to us through OXFAM's refusal to speak well of us to other interested organizations. Ugly as the acceptance of this deal would be, Carl had to think first of the patients who needed a medical service of any kind, and finally agreed upon drawing up a qualified acceptance of Mr. Betts's proposals.

Back at Masianokeng, continuing with our work, the petty irritants seem almost relaxants. We've been out of coffee for two days now, and simply cannot obtain it. I can't stand the taste of tea, so have been doing quite happily without my cup of energy. The doctor says I don't drink tea because I'm just an anti-British snob from America, and though the fact is that the stuff just makes me sick with its perfumed taste, my inability to swallow often makes British social situations difficult.

Poor Rosalia is desperately upset over there being no coffee for me, despite the fact that I hardly give a damn. Despite my protests, she keeps bringing me tea whenever she brings Carl his, and I feel guilty refusing—and can't convince her that I don't like it. Finding my cup always full, she just shakes her head sorrowfully and feels miserable. This morning when she came in with tea for the doctor, she had placed on the tray with it a cup of boiling water. She said hopefully, 'Jeff, wouldn't you like a cup of boiling water? *Ho moruru*, it's a raw day.' Boiling water never tasted so good.

Carl has come down with a high fever and all the symptoms of Asian flu, which has been striking a few people here. Today he still isn't rid of it, partly because he has been working as hard as ever instead of staying in bed.

When I went into his room one evening to see how he was feeling, I found him surrounded on the bed by Suzy, the cat, suckling three screaming kittens; Charles, the doctor's small dog, looking completely baffled and sniffing at the kittens; and Boitjke, the doctor's Alsatian, lying across the whole lot trying to get the doctor's attention. Together we watched these goings on, until Carl commented quietly that if we could get the members of the committee, the government officials, and the missionaries to simply enjoy such a scene our problems would be solved.

We flew to Mafisa the other day. Carl seemed in the morning to be almost over his flu, and felt it safe to fly. But as we were leaving the ground at Masianokeng, Carl yelled back to me, 'No brakes.' One of the big new balloon tyres had crept on its rim, nearly breaking the valve; the tyres are so big, and develop so much leverage when the plane is straining against the brakes, that they creep around the rims. We flew directly to Maseru, landing safely into the wind on the long strip without brakes; we had the smaller tyres put on the plane, and when we removed the bigger tyres found the rim adapters—used to attach the big wheels to the small rims—cracked in about ten different places.

We arrived at Mafisa after a horrendous flight through smoky, blinding clouds, and rode to the clinic from the strip, taking a rowboat across the flooded river while the horses swam.

When we came to the clinic, Carl went directly to work with

his patients and I went to the house to see Helen and John West. I found Helen in the living-room; she really is a lovely, warm woman. Now, however, she looks all worn out and unhappy; when John came in from the shop I learned why.

He greeted me pleasantly, and then immediately flew into a tirade about the 'monkeys' he has to live with. His latest story is that the local court owes him one pound and refuses to give it up to him unless he sends them a letter of request. He refuses to send such a letter because in the past it was necessary to simply have his messenger sign for the money. The pound is owed to him by a starving old woman he sued for a shopping bill she hadn't paid.

He continued his tirade, saying, 'To hell with these monkeys—I don't even speak with them any more. I'm starting an engineering course by mail and then I'm not even going to leave this house to go to the shop; I'm just going to close myself up in this house and study, and in three years I'm leaving this bloody place . . .' Poor Helen just looked on helplessly, and occasionally interjected meekly, 'Really, John, can't you talk about something more pleasant?'

This obsession of his has him in a dangerous position. When I commented on the explosiveness of his present relationship with the local people, he answered angrily, 'When they come to set my house on fire, I'm going out with my shotgun blazing!'

Later, when Carl came in, John went through the same bit again, and Carl just remarked, 'John, can't you find something new to talk about this week to keep things interesting?' John went on, getting deeper into his madness as if there were a purpose in doing so, saying, 'My God, I'd like to grab one of these bastards and just bash his head against the ground, over and over again!'

Flying back from Mafisa to Masianokeng, we got caught in a storm—a huge black storm which reached down all around us with twisting fingers of darkness. The heavy mass of clouds doesn't roll through the sky, but travels with a spider's movement, projecting grotesque fingers ahead of its body. Tossed about by the winds, hardly in control of the plane, we tried to escape from its web, but failed and became prisoners in a cage of twisting black bars. It was as if nature were playing cruel games with us.

We felt as ants must feel when toyed with by a sadistic or viciously curious child.

Much later, upon landing in Maseru, we found the hangars closed and locked. We tied the plane down as best we could and, hoping that it wouldn't blow away in the wind, headed for home.

Having heard rumours of a smallpox epidemic at a village near Khubetsoana, this morning we had to ride to Maseru on the back of a truck, climb into the aeroplane, and fly into what looked like impossible weather conditions. The pilots at the aerodrome in Maseru had told us that flight was unthinkable—there were storm clouds all over the place—but we decided to go up and have a closer look. We found it windy, but not impossible, so entered the mountains through a valley. As we crossed the mountains towards Khubetsoana, we found the weather not only windy, but gusty, and to make things worse the clouds were forcing us to fly right next to the mountains. We were thrown about mercilessly and at one point the plane was tossed up and the engine stalled to a dead silence. Carl dived down, started the prop again, and to our relief a few minutes later Khubetsoana came into sight below us.

We landed on the new airstrip, without the help of a windsock, having to come in crabwise because of a strong crosswind. We couldn't circle around and feel out the wind for it was so powerful and gusty that it kept the plane from turning. We touched down, bounced high into the air, and continued in such a pattern to the end of the strip where we managed to halt.

We spent some time with Molefi, who was starved for company, and we sent for Chief Thaba. When the chief arrived we discussed plans and decided that in two weeks there should be a large feast at the site to officially open the hospital; the doctor will then start working there regularly, with proper patient accommodations. The chief was very friendly, understands perfectly the self-help idea, and will assist us at the time of the feast to choose a clinic committee by popular vote.

At the end of the interview, the chief apologized that he had no money with him, but said he wanted to be examined and would bring the money next week. Carl told him that the chiefs get free treatment, but Chief Thaba says he wants to join the other people in donating towards their hospital.

The smallpox epidemic turned out to be a rumour and little more. In mid-afternoon we took off, but finding the wind gustier than ever, dropped notes to the dispensers at Mohokare and Likhoiting and headed for home. It was a harrowing flight, which took us over three times the normal time because we had to fight the winds all the way.

Two days ago the doctor first flew at sunrise to Khubetsoana again to drop off the builder, Mr. van Jaarsveld, who will put linings in the hospital huts; then he flew to Mohokare to check a new airstrip before going to Mafisa to do a clinic. On the way home from Mafisa late in the day, he dropped a message at Sehlabeng saying that Nurse Mini and I would soon be coming, then stopped briefly at Machache, and finally got caught in a storm and became lost. Before he dropped off to drugged sleep back at Masianokeng he told me excitedly, 'Wherever we go now people come pouring from their homes, the schools, the fields. There are thousands waiting for medical help, wherever we land the countryside is black with people.'

Despite all difficulties, our mountain programme is under way and our spirits high.

March 30 —May 3, 1963

Just after the doctor flew off to the north this morning, Nurse Mini and I went to the Maseru aerodrome to go by charter plane to Sehlabeng where the second hospital unit is to go up. To our surprise, we found that Harry Trident was to fly the plane instead of Myers, the regular Sehlabeng pilot. He did pretty well for his first try, but our nerves suffered none the less.

A huge crowd gathered on the strip as we unloaded the plane, and Morena Pita, our friend Chief, came over to greet us. The people had really begun to doubt that we would ever return.

Amid much confusion, we set up the tent and arranged for Mini to find a better place to stay. Chief insisted on lending her his own hut, saying he will move in with relatives until there is a home built for Mini, and despite our embarrassed protests he refused to hear of any other arrangement. We made coffee in the tent, and Mini, Chief, the old man (who now reeks of alcohol at nine in the morning), and I sat talking. We arranged that Chief would find a man to guide me to Mantsonyane tomorrow, where I must make plans for land transport of the prefabricated buildings—which, because of their being overweight, we cannot afford to have flown in. On the way to Mantsonyane we will stop at the home of the Sehlabeng area chief, Chief Tatolo, to speak with him about building the hospital. Chief insists on lending me his own horse for the trip.

It was kind of difficult at first seeing Chief again, for time had forced some restraint between us, but we trusted each other almost immediately and gradually warmed up again.

Mini said while we were talking that she didn't like this place—

that it's too cold and barren, being on top of a mountain instead of somewhere in a valley. Chief answered that this is a good place because 'Here we plough *dagga*.' *Dagga* is marijuana. Chief went on to say that if he were in the lowlands or in an easily accessible valley he wouldn't be able to plough *dagga*, but here no one stops the people from growing many fields of it. He looked at me with a twinkle in his eye, and we knew that in saying something so daring before me, an outsider, he had broken down the barriers, had again accepted me into his village.

Now I'm sitting in the tent, as it sways in the wind, and squeezed in with me are eleven children. They came to the door and stared under and between the flaps with astonishment when I turned on our new radio, and now, having flexible imaginations, they have already calmed down and are sitting about studying the typewriter and munching sweets we brought with us.

It bothered me last time I was here to have all these kids squirming about, but it doesn't any longer. I used to feel it necessary to pay constant attention to them, and used to feel self-conscious with their staring at me, but now I realize it is fine to just continue with my work and enjoy their spirited presence.

Now Mini has come in and for the past hour the kids have been singing and dancing outside. What a tremendous pleasure it is to watch them. Little innocent kids.

While we were setting up the tent before, we watched a horse-race on the airstrip. The people of the village gathered, the women making high bird-like sounds ('li, li, li, li, li') in admiration of the racing men; the men rode against each other proudly and swiftly on the airstrip. This Sehlabeng village is a rare place—full of a spirit which I haven't met anywhere else in the country. It's wonderful to be back.

When we first stepped off the plane and began getting organized, everyone was staring at us coldly and confusedly, and for a moment I felt just miserable. Then I began to feel even more upset because of the very fact that coming back had made me miserable. But now that we're settled in, and the people are warming up, I feel free and relaxed as I haven't felt since I left this remote village months ago.

The chieftain system here is complicated. To explain it as I understand it: the chief of the Sehlabeng district, the top man, is Morena Tatolo; his brother, Tara Tatolo, is the District Councillor, supposedly representing this district for the government; under the area chief are the village chiefs, such as Chief Tsoelike of the village Ha Tsoelike, Chief Lepolesa of our village Ha Lepolesa, and so on. Each village chief appoints a headman, such as our friend 'Chief' Morena Pita, who is headman under Chief Lepolesa.

Chief lent me his horse for the trip to Mantsonyane, and a man named Moromong agreed to come with me first to see Chief Tatolo and then to ride on to arrange transport of the building materials for Sehlabeng hospital—materials which are now sitting there at the end of the mountain road. We left here at eight in the morning.

We rode quickly to Chief Tatolo's village, slightly out of the way from the shorter route to Mantsonyane; we were told upon our arrival that the chief was in the church. We sat on the ground outside the church to wait, and listened to the lovely singing coming from within.

While we waited, numerous people came out of the church to greet us, and when the chief came I spoke with him for five minutes before I learned that he was in fact Chief Tatolo. He doesn't look very chiefly, but rather is a short man with beady eyes and a pudgy face; he didn't act very friendly, but was sullen and withdrawn. Worried that at the rate things were proceeding we wouldn't get to Mantsonyane before dark, we made an appointment with the chief for Wednesday. The meeting we had was rather solemn, everyone speaking in hushed voices—perhaps because of the church atmosphere.

As we rode off I began to develop saddle sores and to feel the stiffness of riding hard after not having been on a horse for a long time. The weather was beautiful all morning and the going was lovely; we stopped at a stream and ate a few mealies which Moromong had brought, dipped our faces in the icy water, and then continued. By midday the weather began to grow stormy, and the riding was becoming excruciating; my stiff muscles were easily bearable, but the skin was gone from my thighs and my calves were rapidly becoming raw from the rubbing of the stirrup leathers. Storms built up all around us, but somehow never upon us; we could see the valleys filling up with the blackness as we rode through them, the storm dropping its dark and twisting pillars around us, but by riding like mad we managed to get out of each valley before hell broke loose within.

At one point we met on the trail five horsemen—called 'warriors' when they ride in packs—and galloped furiously with them for almost an hour before outdistancing them; later we met some men from our village who were slowly leading a caravan of donkeys to Mantsonyane.

As we rode into the valley of Mantsonyane, we passed a young man fishing in the stream, and his eyes nearly popped out; how mysterious to him are the mountains beyond the end of the mountain road! It was just as if he had watched us ride out of another time dimension into his.

Reaching the new Anglican hospital, our horses weary and ourselves no better for wear, we were met in a friendly manner by Dr. Luckman. We spoke with him for a moment, and he apologized that he had no accommodation because of the campers staying with him; we agreed to meet the next morning as I had some business to discuss with him.

We trudged on to the trader's home where we found that he also had a house full of people, but he lent us two blankets (Moromong, intelligently, had brought his own blankets with him, but not I.) Quite lost, not knowing where to go, and darkness approaching rapidly with a rumbling storm close behind, we went to see Mr. Seabata—the man in charge of the trader's depot. He greeted us warmly and rigged up in the depot beds of baled wool and burlap sacks, which though smelly and not free of rats were relievingly comfortable. I declined an offer of dinner and fell immediately to sleep, just as the storm hit with full force—the wind blowing wildly through the corrugated-iron depot.

I awoke in the morning stiff and aching, and had a rude shock when I got up. My thighs were raw meat, and my underwear edges had dug deeply under the skin. I washed, had a cup of coffee with Seabata—who was wonderful to us—while Moromong, who had risen much earlier, went to get the horses. Seabata and I discussed at length the transport of the building materials. I learned that there is no chance of getting transport for under fifty pounds and that we would be lucky to get that low an offer at this time of year. It is harvesting season, and the donkeys are all being used in the fields; also, the men who do transporting from Mantsonyane to various other mountain shops make money on the return trip too, while in this case they would be bringing unloaded donkeys back to Mantsonyane. If the people of Sehlabeng want a hospital, they will have to transport the stuff themselves. They certainly should be willing to do so, and we will give them as a gesture of thanks thirty or so pounds from the small amount remaining in our mountain fund.

I walked the mile to the hospital, leaving a message for Moromong to meet me there, and was met at the gate by Dr. Luckman. We sat and talked for a while; I suggested something Carl and I had been discussing for some time: the idea that all the doctors throughout the country pitch into mountain work, each giving one day out of every two weeks, with us offering them the use of the aeroplane. Dr. Luckman didn't like the idea a bit; he said, 'It's dangerous . . . there are no good facilities for emergency operations in the mountains anyway . . .' I restrained myself. It all boils down, I think, to the fact that he doesn't like the idea of flying, and that's certainly understandable.

What irritated me was the way he views our work. He spoke as if I were here on vacation and Carl flying the plane around the mountains for kicks. I wonder whether he has any conception of the horrible situation in the more remote spots in the mountains. I told myself, perhaps we expect too much of people, and kept quiet. It's true—we do expect too much of people, and have no right to.

Apart from our own pain of getting on the horses for the return trip, there was the cruelty of not letting the horses rest any length of time. They were really exhausted and out of the commonest decency we should have given them a day, preferably two days, rest. The problem is that Chief needed his horse back right away, and lent it to me on that basis; he wouldn't understand my ideas about decency to animals as an excuse for not returning his horse on time. The treatment of animals by even the nicest local people is appalling, a difficult thing to confront. The horses are trained to move when beaten, so that anyone who wishes to get anywhere must strike his horse whether or not he believes in such treatment of animals. If the horse is borrowed, it must be treated as the owner demands; if you insist on letting the horse rest and the owner therefore doesn't get it back in the time he wishes, you just mustn't borrow the horse in the first place; the owner can't understand compassion for the beast as a reason why he must walk instead of ride to his fields the next day.

Numerous times on the way home I felt that I should have had the courage to tell Moromong that we must stop, that we must let the horses rest for at least a day, that we must at least ride slowly even if we are inconvenienced by arriving home after dark, but I knew that he wouldn't hear me. Chief wanted his horse back, and Moromong wanted to get home to his wife before she should go to another man. Still, I felt guilty, and couldn't reconcile myself to the necessity of treating the animal so brutally. When we stopped briefly for various reasons, I rubbed the horse's forehead and it nuzzled me as if I were treating it kindly—which made me feel worse.

The trip to Mantsonyane had been painful, but the trip home to Sehlabeng was indescribable torture. Just as I was beginning to get numb, it started to pour and the rain was freezing cold—lightning was everywhere and the trails were fearfully slippery. Moromong gave me one of his blankets to wear, and I rode along looking and feeling like a Mosotho. I couldn't smoke because my fingers were numb, my pants and saddle were soaked and the chafing on my sores was blindingly painful; the horses were slipping on the fresh mud so that we never knew whether they might fall and send us careening down a mountainside.

It's odd how one's moods shift on such a trip, throughout such an experience. Through much of it I felt that I just could not go on for another minute, much less for the many hours ahead, yet knew that I must somehow do it and went on and on. Yet, there were moments of just the opposite feeling, a feeling of supreme elation, which despite their fleeting nature were worth it all.

As we rode, many people recognized us, and at one point a group of about ten women stood on the side of the trail shouting and cheering as we rode past; one came to us and said that her baby had been very ill and that she would bring it to the nurse tomorrow.

When we rode through a small village only a couple of hours from home, a man and his wife stopped us and insisted that we come into their hut for food. We were starved, and entered their smoke-filled hut, stooping to the floor for air to breathe. Moromong and I were glad for the warmth of the fire and the goodness of these people. The wife went out after she had helped us settle in the hut, and brought back a whole pint of milk which she had just worked from her cow; she heated it on the fire, and gave it to us with two heaping plates of corn meal. In our exhausted state, we drank the warm milk, and felt like helpless children before her kindness.

We rode towards our village by a seldom-used trail, through a deep valley lush and untouched. We went along the side of a stream, under a waterfall, and into reeds which were at least ten feet tall. Blinded by the reeds which brushed around us, we were surrounded by a world of sounds: the chirping of birds which scattered furiously at our approach. Then we suddenly came out of the reed world into fields of a coarse plant about four feet high which smelled overpoweringly of mint. The horses had a grand time, snatching off great mouthfuls of this minty plant as they continued their pace and Moromong and I grinned at each other like kids, elated in this paradise.

The mountain climb up to the village was so steep and the poor horses so tired that we walked them up the rocky slope until we were about to collapse from exhaustion. We took the horses to Chief's hut where he insisted on taking care of them for us, seeing that we were nine-tenths dead.

I sighed with relief, and set off in the dark for the tent, about a quarter mile distant. I somehow managed to get totally lost. I was completely blinded, having just ridden through dusk, and must have taken a wrong turn somewhere. Weak and frustrated almost to tears, I walked and walked until I found a hut with people about, and a woman there showed me back to Chief's place, keeping her distance from me as if I were a madman. I was much too tired to rape her. Chief immediately saw my condition, and took me back to the tent himself; instead of coming inside as usual to chat, he told me as a father might that I must go straight to sleep and that he would see me in the morning.

I swallowed a mug of brandy to overcome the exhaustion which was about to make me vomit, and as I crawled into the sleeping bag the old man came to the door to ask whether I was all right. I lit the candle and spoke with him for a few minutes, and noticed that he was staring at me strangely. I looked at my hand,

and found it covered with blood—from having touched sores I had in my numbness forgotten. The skin was torn completely away from my legs, leaving hundreds of bleeding sores.

It was a long time before I found sleep. My head reeled with gratitude, gratitude for being home again, and gratitude for the kindness of the people around me. I could hardly cope with it, and the loneliness I felt.

This morning I awoke late to find the sun shining, the tent hot and full of flies, many of which had settled on my lips which were cracked from the sun and wind.

Now once again, I have a tent full of children; they just sit and stare, asking questions once in a while about this or that object. When I look directly at any one of them, he grins with a beam the likes of which exist nowhere else.

Nurse Mini spent yesterday cleaning out the hut which we have been using for storage, and it looks like a new place. The rats which used to live in the straw that littered the floor have been pushed up to the roof, and the hut looks habitable. Medicines are sitting on improvised tables around the walls, and even with a stretcher in the little hut there is enough room to work. The old man who owns the place is amazed, and so am I. It took a woman to do it.

The people here have been treating us wonderfully; every morning the woman in the hut next door calls me to her hut and gives me a big jug of beer (which I gratefully force down—ugh), and when a woman from another village came to sell us potatoes, a group of people from this village told her angrily that we should not pay—that our work is a service for the people and that we shouldn't have to pay for being here.

This morning there are thirty patients to see Nurse Mini, and as people get used to her there will be many more coming. She is highly qualified, has had much experience, is a registered midwife, and can supplement her abilities with the help of the patients' record sheets accumulated by Carl. Her work shows that a clinic with such a highly qualified staff-nurse/midwife and a dispenser is effective and efficient as a medical service, though certainly far from the ideal set-up of having a permanent or regularly visiting doctor. If such a mountain clinic had a doctor on call for emergencies, however, it would be quite close to ideal.

I was able to sleep for only a few hours last night, and those were fitful. I kept imagining that something had happened to the doctor, with all the flying he's doing this week. I had the morbid feeling that a message was about to arrive telling us of an accident. I've been with this ugly train of thought ever since I spoke with Dr. Luckman at Mantsonyane who said, 'He can't go on like this forever; while he does he will be doing more than anyone else here, but he is bound to wreck that plane and kill himself before long.' There's much truth in that statement, for in flying nearly every day of the week—and when exhausted and worried by various difficulties—Carl is piling up the odds against himself. I worry also that he is not one hundred per cent pilot, but rather is all doctor, flying sometimes as a doctor when a pilot would refuse to fly.

I was visited today by Tara Tatolo, the District Councillor. He is a tall, handsome man, very intelligent and seemingly a fine person. We had some coffee, and discussed where would be the best place to build. He was undecided whether we should build at this site, or at Ha Tsoelike, a village closer to his and Chief Tatolo's home. He is pleased with our ideas about self-help, and is anxious to do all he can to help us reach the people. He says he has no doubt that the people here will be readily willing to bring the materials from Mantsonyane and help build the hospital. He wants to help form a local committee just as soon as we choose a hospital site.

After we had spoken together for half an hour, Morena Tatolo, the area chief, came in—after riding over three hours here in the rain. Chief Tatolo's looks and personality are certainly not in keeping with his respectful position. He is just like a little boy, spoiled and obstinate, yet lovable. When I began to explain to him what Tara Tatolo and I had just been discussing, saying, 'The problem is whether to build here or at Ha Tsoelike . . .' he interrupted insistently, 'Come to Ha Tsoelike, nearer to my home.' I reacted with surprise, and a look which said, 'It is not so simple,' but seeing the pout I had produced by my failure to instantly agree with him, I had to laugh. We discussed the matter for a long time, and to combat the cold weather, had some brandy. He ignores all rationality, and persists with pure selfishness, all the time giving you a look, a childish look, which says,

'I know I'm being a stubborn brat, but I'm a chief and I can get away with it.' The fact that we cannot possibly build at Ha Tsoelike unless we find it possible to level an airstrip there means nothing to him. He WANTS us to build nearer to his home.

We finally agreed to meet at Ha Tsoelike on Friday—he will send a horse for me—to take a look at the proposed site. We will get the people to work on the possible airstrip, and when the doctor comes he will try landing on the strip to see if it is OK. If the strip is better than the one here, we will build at Ha Tsoelike. The site is somewhat in a river valley rather than at the top of the mountain, therefore providing more fertile land and better weather conditions. If the strip isn't practical, we build here at Ha Lepolesa—a decision of necessity, remote from Chief Tatolo's whims.

I'm impressed by Chief Tatolo's strange sort of candour, and also by the fact that he has on his own been calling numerous *pitsos* to lecture the people on self-help. Tara Tatolo is a more mature and unselfish individual, but is somehow too mild for strong, decisive action.

While the chiefs were here, there were over a hundred persons come, despite the rain, to see Nurse Mini for medical treatment. One man came into the tent after Chief Tatolo had left to ask for work; as soon as I looked at him, I was startled—there was something cruelly bitter about his look, and a strength in it of frightening reality. Then I noticed that he had a wooden leg; he told me that a witch-doctor had amputated his leg a few years ago and that he had been unable to get work since—that he and his family are starving. I told him that I would give him work at the hospital site, and he was overwhelmed with surprise. The hard bitterness in his face cleared with remarkable alacrity, though his strength of character softened not at all. We sat there together in silence for nearly half an hour before he thanked me and took leave.

Yesterday afternoon I worked at the dispensary with Mini (we were inundated with patients); when I came back to the tent I found that someone had dug a ditch around it to keep the rain waters from running in. I still haven't found out which good person did it.

Later I went to the edge of the village to take a picture of the sunset with some colour film I'm trying for the first time. A woman saw me taking the photo and came over to ask if I would take a picture of her. I didn't want to because the colour film is so costly, but she was so excited that I couldn't tell her no. As soon as I had agreed, twenty women came running and lined up expectantly. As I raised the camera to take the picture, all the women suddenly threw off their blankets, baring their breasts while I took the photo. Immediately after, they covered themselves. At least the superficial niceties of our society are imposed only shallowly on these beautiful people.

I had to spend the later part of the afternoon in the dispensary giving injections not so much because Mini didn't have time in which to do it herself, but because I was in popular demand. A large group of women had got together in protest of my not being the one to inject their medicines; the reason was, in their words, that unlike Mini I give 'respectful injections'. Mini gives all injections in the rear end while I usually prefer to inject people in the arm.

In the evening, as Mini and I were again cooking chips for dinner, Chief came in. I asked him if he likes chips, and he didn't know what I was talking about. When I gave him one from the first batch we had just finished frying, he tasted it carefully and said, 'Ummm, I like it.' After chewing it for a moment, he said thoughtfully, 'It tastes like some pork I once had.' He stayed with us for supper.

I told him that he should put a lot of salt on chips, and began to pour salt on his plate. But he gave a start, and quickly stopped me, saying, 'If I use so much salt I'll commit rape and have to go to jail.' I asked him what the hell he was talking about, and he explained that the people know that salt and eggs in large quantities make one commit rape. All through dinner, whenever I put some salt on my chips, he warned me seriously that I'd better tie myself down in the tent for the night, or he would have to put me in jail the next day.

We talked for a while about the mission, and about the priest's continued unfriendliness. Chief said that the priest had told many people that if they come to our clinic they had better not come to his church. His words have become softer. Chief doesn't call the mission '*missione*' as do the other people here, but because the priest is from Quebec, he points to the mission and calls it

'Canada'. He said he would lend me his horse on which to go to Canada if I wished, but that he himself wouldn't go near 'the wild Canadian'.

The chief claims he doesn't know any English, and I think he's telling the truth. I had suspected that he secretly did, but it turns out that the few words he does know are those he learned in the South African mines. He says he knows the words 'come on' because that's what the bosses in the mines used to yell when they kicked him and the other workers. When he's on his horse, he can be heard yelling, 'Come on, come on!' instead of the usual '*eeee-yaaah!*'

This morning a charter plane flew over, despite bad winds, and dropped a note. In great anxiety we searched for the message and couldn't find it, until finally some man started yelling that he had come across it. It turned out to be good news, not bad, much to our relief. Carl had written that the clinics at Khubetsoana, Mohokare, and Likhoiting have been huge successes, that the people at Khubetsoana have agreed to transport their hut linings from Mantsonyane, and that the people at Bobeti keep insisting that if the villagers of Sehlabeng are reluctant to transport their five buildings from Mantsonyane, their people will take them and build them themselves at Likhoiting. That should be a good spur to the people here at Sehlabeng.

Carl is coming here on Monday to see patients—weather permitting.

Yesterday, despite rotten weather, a man showed up from Ha Tsoelike with an extra horse for me and we rode off to choose a site and get people working on the airstrip. When we were about halfway there it started to pour, but we ignored the rain; since Carl had sent a note saying that he is coming Monday, it was necessary for us to rush with the strip. The ride was rather painful, what with freezing rain, old saddle sores opening, and slippery trails. When we reached Ha Tsoelike, Tara Tatolo, Chief Tatolo, and Chief Tsoelike were waiting for us and we went despite the rain to have a look around and make a decision.

We looked at the potential airstrip the doctor had had in mind, but found it just terrible—requiring months of work to smooth the land at all. Also, it has many disadvantages as a site; it is far from the river, and located on a plateau which can be reached only by one trail.

Chief Tsoelike, a sleepy-looking old man with wire-rimmed spectacles, said that he had an idea for a place, but since we had never mentioned it he figured it was no good. I told him that was lousy reasoning, and he took us there. It is beautiful, a huge plateau, and the trails from every village in the area cross right by it. It is surrounded on three sides by the river, and offers a place for a strip which would be right next to an expansive building site. The strip is smooth, hardly needing any work at all, and though it is only two hundred yards long it is very steeply inclined. Most of our too short airstrips are three or four hundred yards long; if the strip is inclined as is this one, however, the Cub can land take off in less than a hundred yards. I was excited about the place, and the chiefs readily agreed that if the plane can land there we can have for our use the plateau, and, if we like, some of the mealie lands nearby for community farming work.

My only worry about the strip is that a high ridge across the base might be in the way of landing and take-off, but that's to be seen. I suppressed my excitement in order that we shouldn't later have to disappoint everyone if the strip is no good.

The people are now filling in the few holes there are in the ground, and a man who owns a small shop nearby is lending us pieces of corrugated iron for temporarily marking the strip so that Carl can spot it from the air. On Monday morning the doctor will try it; when they hear the plane the people at Ha Tsoelike will light a large fire to indicate the wind direction.

As it was late in the day by the time we had finished marking off the land, and the rain was still pouring down, I agreed to ride to Ha Lepolesa alone and let someone pick up the horse the next day. The idea bothered me because the trails were in such dangerous condition, but I did feel like riding alone, choosing my own pace for a change, and didn't want to make anyone ride unnecessarily in the rain to Ha Lepolisa, a few hours away.

After fifteen minutes of riding, the rain finally ended and the sun came out, immediately pulling me out of a low mood. I took a long route through the valley, going beside the streams which were roaring after the rain, and spent about ten minutes in a forest of thirty lonely trees in which the noise of birds seemed deafening. I travelled through some villages Molefi and I used to visit and saw many old friends who hadn't known I was back. They came running out of their huts as I went by and spoke with me elatedly. It was a lovely ride, except for the mud which was splattering all over me and threatening to make the horse slip. The whole trip was like a fantasy: everything seemed to awake as the sun came out and huge rainbows spanned the valleys; the mist, left hanging just above the ground, felt delicate on my face as I rode through it, its light beads bursting against my skin; and the woollen hat I was wearing radiated that wonderful musty smell wool has when the sun dries it.

When I arrived back in our village Chief came out to help me with my horse, and while I changed from my muddy clothes he took it to the fields to graze for the night. He was surprised that I had ridden home alone, and asked with a twinkle, 'Weren't you afraid of being eaten?' I laughed, but he said, now with serious concern, 'Don't you know that chiefs eat people? Chief Lepisa of the nearby village you rode through eats many people.'

Later, while we were having dinner, I asked Chief to again show me the fountain near by our village. He said, 'I thought you had decided to build at Ha Tsoelike.' I answered that we might, but aren't sure yet, that the people at Ha Tsoelike want us to build there, but we will do so only if it seems to be the best place for a hospital. That's why I wished to again see the local site—so that I can compare it with the one at Ha Tsoelike. Chief said angrily that it is stupid the way people insist that we build in their village—that such thinking can only cause fights. He realizes that we are concerned with practical considerations like airstrips and water supply. He then said that we should build wherever we think best, and that the chiefs would see that everybody in every nearby village co-operates—for the hospital is for everyone in the area. He would like to see us build there for selfish reasons, but would rather see us establish the hospital where it can do the most good; if we are building at Ha Tsoelike, he still will do everything he can to help us.

As we were finishing dinner, a gigantic storm started rolling toward Sehlabeng; Mini and Chief retreated to their homes for the night. What a storm it was! All night the tent was blown about and the rain lashed it with frightening force. Fortunately

I had in the afternoon rigged up a pole in the middle of the tent for added strength, and perhaps it was for that reason that the tent didn't blow away. For all the protection the canvas gave me, however, it might as well have blown away; the pounding rain was so powerful that it came through the fabric in a fine, freezing spray. I crawled deep into the sleeping bag to get away from it, and when I awoke this morning everything in the tent, including the pillow and myself, was soaked through.

It's still raining now in the same manner, and when it slows down we can hear the river, miles away, roaring as if it were at our feet.

The rain continued all yesterday morning, and finally let up for a bit at about two in the afternoon. The weather remained bitter and raw, but a bunch of children—about thirty of them—came and, despite the cold, danced and sang near the tent. Mini and I went out to watch and hear them and for about an hour were so warmed by their spirit that we forgot the cold. What a sight—I wish I could describe it: in this bleak weather, the barren mountains more desolate than ever, these children, some dressed in ragged blankets, other in only burlap sacks for clothing, sang and danced together with a gaiety unmatchable.

When the rain had again started, and was pouring through the tent as ever, Chief came to say that he remembered another tent, a ripped one, which the doctor had used the first time he was here. We searched through our stuff in the dispensary hut and found it—ripped, but a good deal larger than the present tent. Chief and I went out in the rain to rig it up over my little tent, stretching it tight to form large air pockets between the canvases. It served its purpose perfectly, and I spent a rarely peaceful night.

The doctor couldn't come yesterday because of rain; we expect him today or tomorrow. This visit will now be mostly to choose the final site, for there probably won't be many patients; the rivers are flooded and impossible to cross, so the patients have no way of getting here. Even those patients who don't have to cross rivers will have difficulty on slippery trails.

Nurse Mini, however, has seen hundreds of patients, and there was only one whose illness was not readily diagnosable. Here the commonest diseases are the worst killers. The local people are extremely pleased with Mini; people in the village tell us that everyone is saying the doctor has sent them good people, that now he is really providing a service for them upon which they can depend.

There have been ceremonies here almost every night; as soon as darkness comes, drums start beating, and throughout the whole night they keep on. Chief tells me that this week the witch-doctors go from hut to hut all night warning certain people of what fate has in store for them. The *ngakas* can tell people when they must watch out for poison and such witchcraft.

Last night, at about sunset, it became, as always, freezing cold. The old man came into our tent, and began lecturing us about how we must build a fire in the tent (the people all build fires in their huts—the smoke of burning dung becoming so thick that it's nearly impossible to breathe). I explained to him that the tarpaulin on the floor would catch fire, and he said adamantly, 'Then you must roll it back.' He was furious at the idea of our being cold, and went on in this manner for nearly an hour. Finally he dragged us into his own hut and made us sit by the fire.

Later, Chief came to dinner. We love having him here and he comes even if he is not hungry for dinner, partly because he likes our company as we like his, also because he doesn't want Mini to walk alone to her hut at night and protests against my taking her because it's so cold and I don't wear a warm blanket as he does.

We are often visited by a lovely girl here of about twenty or twenty-one. She's really charming, a person who is either delighted to the degree of forgetting to be shy or embarrassed to the point of being completely tongue-tied—and she's so pretty that one can't help but enjoy her presence. Yesterday she entered the dispensary hut with a display of timidity unusual even from her, and hastily presented me with about ten cobs of corn she carried in a bag. When I expressed my pleasure at the gift, she broke into great smiles of relief. Mini later told me that the girl had come to her to ask if I liked mealies; Mini, not being sure, said that I probably did. The girl was frightened that perhaps I wouldn't like them, and had sat for over an hour trying to decide whether to take a chance and offer them to me.

Carl was unable to land the plane at Sehlabeng because of the land's swampiness after the torrential rains; also the flying conditions were impossible because of heavy mist hanging blindingly over the valleys. Late in the afternoon he flew over and dropped a note, saying abruptly, 'Weather conditions unsuitable; come down via Mantsonyane.' Mini and I saw immediately that something was wrong, and we began trying to figure how I could manage to get to Mantsonyane the next day—it being difficult if not impossible to get horses at such short notice, and quite a dangerous trick to cross the rivers in flood.

We found Moromong, and he agreed to take me there again though it was clear that the idea displeased him; we insisted that he take payment as thanks from us, although he was genuinely reluctant to accept it. We then found Chief, who said without hesitation that if it were important for me to go he would lend me his horse. We made preparations for the trip.

On Thursday morning, just before sunrise, Chief arrived at my tent with his saddled horse, and after loading the saddle bags, we had coffee in the tent. Moromong showed up a few minutes later, and we set off in the early morning's darkness in the hope of arriving at Mantsonyane in time for me to catch a lift that day to Masianokeng. Before we left, Moromong, remembering the pains I had suffered last time, slung an extra blanket over the saddle of my horse.

We rode hard, fast as is possible on these murderous trails, and were threatened throughout the ride by storm clouds. Finally the threat became a reality and we were thoroughly soaked and frozen by the time Mantsonyane came into sight. We arrived there at two-thirty in the afternoon, and though I wasn't this time stiff or raw, I was exhausted to the point of collapse. Even Moromong looked more dead than alive, and headed for the village to find a sleeping place.

We had met no one on the trail during the ride, probably because of the weather conditions and high rivers. We had had to cross Mantsonyane River in flood, on horseback; the horses were swimming rather than walking, and the water was above our hips. Numerous times the rapid waters nearly carried us away—but, carefully avoiding thoughts of the churning, rocky horror downstream from us, we urged the horses on violently and finally gained the other side. Once having made the crossing we realized what fools we were to attempt it.

When my bus from Mantsonyane stopped at Masianokeng and I started for the house, all the boys came running to the road to greet me, Boitjke running excitedly after them. When I entered the kitchen, I was nearly smothered—in such a pleasant way—by Rosalia. I walked through the house and into Carl's room to find him sitting at his desk with his head buried in his hands. He looked up and said, 'My God! It's Jeff, Jeff . . . I've never been so glad to see anyone. We were just going to go and get you with the aeroplane this morning, but it rained and I never thought I'd see you today; I've been in a panic. How are you? How did you get back? Thank goodness you're here!' As I staggered to recover my balance after this most remarkable effusiveness coming from Carl, he ran out of the room and returned with an empty glass which he filled to the brim with brandy—pushing me into a chair and presenting me with this sweet relief.

Carl explained that this very evening of my return the Scotts were expected. The Scotts are the possible administrative couple, old acquaintances of Carl's, who have shown interest for years in joining him here. They have a reputation in the Republic of being extremely capable and liberal people. They in fact arrived the next morning.

The Scotts explained that Betts had sent them a telegram requesting that they see him on the way. Apparently he also was interested in securing their services, and he had in fact offered them a position in Johannesburg with an OXFAM scheme at a salary of three hundred and fifty pounds per month plus a car.

The Scotts stayed as our guests. We spoke extensively with them, through Saturday and into Sunday morning; we argued about how large a role business deserves in our type of work, and discussed the morality of OXFAM's loan to BASOMED. Though we disagreed on many things, that was to be expected. But all in all, the Scotts voiced sympathy for our position. We of course are concerned at the possible connection between OXFAM and the

British government. Independence is due for Bastutoland within the next three years. If the various medical, social, education, and agricultural services of a newly-independent African state are administratively controlled in full by OXFAM, and if OXFAM is too closely linked with British government as indicated by recent developments, and if the African country's businesses are already British owned as indeed they are here, then what is, in fact, the meaning of 'independence'?

The Scotts finally said that they would like to see us succeed as a private organization. We felt that if they would take on the administrative position independently of OXFAM, we might have a chance—and we felt that we had a right to ask them to do so, for Carl knew them and had spoken with them about the idea long before OXFAM entered the picture, but they said that they were embarrassed and did not want to take sides.

Carl has spoken with his accountant in Bloemfontein, who feels that the OXFAM loan, with its present conditions, is a bad risk; on the other hand, he feels that in view of Mr. Betts's having spoken already with our creditors, there would be no chance in the world of holding them off should we reject the loan. He wanted badly to be helpful, but could see no alternative to our accepting the loan and hoping for the best.

We have another possible candidate for administrator. He is from Capetown, and is very interested in the BASOMED position. He is presently applying for a legal exit permit, permanent, from the Republic; we hope he'll be here next week. Betts has already promised him the job with BASOMED, and has assured him of a fifteen hundred pound salary paid directly by OXFAM. We will see him, for he sounds qualified, and may be a man of independent character. In the meantime we continue with our work, which threatens to be forgotten in all this administrative rubble.

Two days ago I flew to Semongkong with Basutair and stayed overnight with the trader there. He found a horse for my eleven-hour trip the next morning to Sehlabeng, and at nine I set off, leading an extra pack-horse loaded with medicines. Surrounded by challenging open country, I quickly left administrative problems behind me.

I arrived long after dark, to find Sehlabeng sound asleep. I was frozen through and sore, my clothes soaked from crossing icy rivers. I took care of the horses, and went off to the tent for blessed sleep.

Shuffling sounds outside the tent this morning hardly disturbed my long sleep. When I finally went out, I found about thirty people standing about waiting to greet me, all whistling in amazement upon my answering their questions as to how I had got here. Mini came and was much relieved; she has been terribly lonely, and by yesterday was frightened that something wrong must have happened to keep me away. She had no medicines for patients all the past week.

People told me that they had known I would return and not let them down, and Mini was in her good way just happy that Carl and I were OK, and that I had brought the badly-needed supplies. She was tickled by a gift of two apples and a few other treats I had furtively slipped into my pockets instead of eating at the Semongkong trader's.

I must begin my return to Masianokeng on Tuesday, arriving there Wednesday night, to be with Carl when he interviews the new administrative applicant, or 'administrator' I guess I must say. Carl says he just cannot talk to new people about the work alone, that he feels embarrassed to the point of reticence having to back up his own cause.

We must now call a *pitso* here at Sehlabeng of people from every village in the district, in order to discuss the final location of the hospital, transport of building materials from Mantsonyane, the reasons for Carl's temporary absence, and the whole concept of the hospital. There seems to be a good spirit among the local people.

Chief and I discussed again the subjects I want to cover at the *pitso*; he was pleased, and had some good suggestions to add. But he feels that if we give the people only short notice, we won't get a very big turnout; it would be best that when I come again from Masianokeng in a week or so we should give good advance notice and draw a large crowd. If there aren't enough people present at the *pitso*, much confusion will result, and besides, we aren't sure yet whether the Ha Tsoelike airstrip is usable and should know for sure before making any definite plans. Of course he was absolutely right.

He added that all I have to do at this time is say '*olokele*', 'OK', and the people will begin transport of the building materials from Mantsonyane; explanations of other things can wait until my return.

I said '*olokele*', and sure enough, a number of people have offered donkeys. Transport starts tomorrow. With the number of donkeys we have, it shouldn't take long at all.

When at the end of our conversation Chief offered his horse for my trip to Mantsonyane, I told him that I feel bad that whenever we need help it is he who makes an offer while the situation should be that everyone gives a bit. I wondered whether I could do anything for him personally, like bringing him something from Maseru when I return. He said that he is only too happy to help, and that I mustn't thank him—that it is he who should thank me. He promised finally that if he needs anything he will let me know, but insisted that I mustn't worry about it. Men such as Chief make everything and anything worthwhile.

Moromong told me on Sunday that he would like to get to Mantsonyane before the donkeys so that he can make sure everything gets packed correctly for transport.

We set off at nine the next morning for Mantsonyane after making sure all the donkeys were ready—nine donkeys to begin with and more joining them, despite the fact that this is harvesting season when donkeys are extremely scarce. I had my first accident on the trip, when my horse slipped on slanting rock formations and my right foot caught in its stirrup; I must have grown overconfident, for if I had been riding properly my foot would have fallen free. Instead I was dragged twenty feet over the rocks by a panicky horse before I got a grip on my senses and loosed my foot from the stirrup. Badly bruised around the back, and bleeding quite heavily from the legs and arms, I felt for broken bones, and finding none, sat there half stunned. Moromong ran over and just stood looking so shocked that when I saw him I could feel only his fear. But it was all right, and after my many lengthy protests that I was unhurt, Moromong finally muttered '*Olokele*', and we rode on, carefully. My horse was in good shape despite his fall.

When we arrived at the Mantsonyane shop depot late in the afternoon, Mr. Seabata greeted us with engulfing warmth and said that he had been hoping we would come in time to enjoy his new facilities. He dragged us into the depot and from its ratty innards produced two huge beds with real mattresses of straw, saying proudly, 'These are being transported soon to the mission at Sebesong, but tonight you will sleep in comfort.' He made the beds while he held us off from helping, and then touched off the works of art with pillows, each consisting of five burlap bags previously used for donkey transport.

As luck would have it, this night was the coldest of the year—the bitterest cold I've ever felt or imagined. We learned later that it had been $-20°$F. Seabata invited us into his hut, where we sat in front of a coal fire, coal being very rare here, and ate sheep's liver, delicious, for dinner.

The next morning, while awaiting a lift to Masianokeng, I spent some time in the Mantsonyane trader's shop for warmth. Any time spent in a mountain shop is a moving experience, and this one typifies the lot. It is a long rectangular building with a large empty room on one end where grain, wool, and other merchandise is weighed; the counter and cash register are in a small, narrow middle room which is actually little more than a corridor into the third room, that being the large, main shop where all sorts of goods are sold. The whole set-up is so constructed that when one comes he goes into the first room to sell his goods to the trader; gets a slip of paper which he carries into the middle room for cash on his way to the shop; and exits from the shop itself. Thus he usually uses the precious money of his sale in buying from the shop.

I have spent hours at Mantsonyane sitting on the long counter in the middle room of the shop, where one can look through a large picture window out into the front yard of the whole complex. One can sit there for hours, watching with horrible fascination, sometimes seeing scenes so sad that one wants to cry.

A common sight is that of a child coming from places over a day or two days' walk away to sell what she has managed to collect over a month of time. You see a little girl about six years old walk onto the shop grounds; she is dressed in only a ragged blanket despite the bitter weather, and she carries a tiny bowl of peas on her head, a bowl so small that it is no larger than a man's cupped hands. She doesn't enter immediately, but stands still, frightened by this new world of 'civilization', watching people enter and leave the shop; she has never seen a shop before—never seen any building but a mud hut. Then she begins the ritual of timidity, starting to enter the shop, then stopping and waiting, then again feinting towards the shop door. Finally, after half an hour or more, she gingerly enters the first door, the little girl of six, overawed by the size of the building and the activity within. The trader sees her enter, swoops into the first room where she stands bewildered, takes from her clutching hands the bowl of peas, and with one flick of his wrist dumps her harvest into a huge sack already three-quarters full. Handing her a scrap of paper in receipt, he retires into the middle room and takes his place behind the counter to wait.

The little girl again stands awkwardly for a few minutes before gathering the courage to enter the middle room and stand before the counter. The trader whisks up her slip of paper, and plonks a penny or twopence—or even threepence, if the number of peas warrant it—on the counter. The child picks up the small coin, and starts for the doorway where she came in—but, the trader stops her, and steers her towards the correct exit, that one leading through the room where the merchandise of the shop is displayed gaudily.

You see the child entering the shop, and a few minutes later watch her step out of the last door carrying a single candle, or a small cake of soap, and now without hesitation she starts her one, or two, or perhaps even three-day walk home.

We arrived at Masianokeng at about five in the afternoon, and Sechlobi, the first of the boys home from school, came out to help me with my meagre baggage and to say hello. I saw sitting in the yard a number of people—the new administrator and his wife, Carl, and Cardwell Mciteka. Carl yelled, 'Look, this must be a mirage,' and came running out to greet me. I assured him that all is fine at Sehlabeng, the building materials being transported, and he told me that things here are not too bad. After introducing me to the guests who had arrived the previous evening, and giving me a moment to exchange warm greetings with Cardwell, he ushered me into the house and insisted that I have some brandy and coffee with him. He is pleased with the first impression of the new administrative couple.

Dinner with the new administrative couple had already been

arranged, and Carl insisted that I come along to fill them in on local details. Apparently he had been saying all afternoon in answer to their questions, 'Jeff will explain when he arrives.'

At dinner I told them of Carl's work and of the country itself—lowlands and mountains—in a most staightforward manner, figuring they might as well know now. They responded with candour. We didn't break up until eleven, and all had a good time. They will be staying at the hotel tonight and moving tomorrow morning to Masianokeng.

Their name is Hoogendyk, Jan and Jacki. Jan feels that while he needs the OXFAM salary, we must not allow BASOMED's principles to go under. As for the OXFAM stipulation that the administrative couple should take over the house, while the doctor should find a new place to stay when in the lowlands, Jan and Jacki feel that they have no right to take over what is so clearly Carl's home. For the time being we will all share it, until Jan and Jacki can find a home of their own. They seem fine people, sensitive and considerate.

Back at Masianokeng Carl and I made the decision to formally accept the OXFAM loan, for the decision cannot be put off any longer. We do so despairingly, but look with hope towards our rapidly-developing mountain work, and are somewhat encouraged by our talks with the new administrators. Together we drew up the necessary memorandum, then went to bed.

May 4 — July 29, 1963

Today we were shattered by news brought by Mr. van Jaarsveld from Mantsonyane, where he had gone to sort out what building materials hadn't yet been transported to Sehlabeng. He came back to tell us that none of the materials have gone, and that the man in charge of the Mantsonyane depot says the donkeys never arrived to his knowledge. We know that the donkeys must have come, for I left Sehlabeng with them. It seems, however, that the men with the donkeys must have taken some other transport job for a high price, donkeys being scarce now in the harvesting season and their services worth a great deal of money to traders. This comes as a great disappointment. Perhaps I put too much faith in people. I had thought that at least things were going well in the mountains, especially at Sehlabeng. I had made preparations to return there.

Arrived here at Sehlabeng yesterday morning on a charter plane, and we were met by an enthusiastic crowd. We found that Molefi Thinyane, who planned to meet us here, had not yet arrived. But we had coffee with Mini, and she explained that a second brigade of donkeys had left three days ago for Mantsonyane; Molefi must have met them on the trail and gone with them to get everything squared up. Mini tells us that when the first group of donkeys went, Moromong had met them at Mantsonyane as planned; when the men with the beasts had looked at the load of building materials, they had refused to transport it because there was so much. Moromong had got furious and said he would drive the donkeys home alone, but the men refused. So, of all the damn things, the donkeys returned carrying nothing. Now, after orders from Chief, this second group of donkeys has gone.

Moromong came from the next village to meet us, and apologized profusely for all the transport difficulties. We thanked him for all his strong efforts, and received his assurance that everyone in the village is upset at the problems; many women have threatened to go and carry the stuff back on their heads if the men won't do the work with donkeys.

Come evening, as Mini, van Jaarsveld, Chief and I were eating supper, we were interrupted by a groaning sound outside. It was Molefi, who literally fell into the tent. He had walked from Mantsonyane, carrying a pile of heavy baggage; no horses had been available for him. It had taken him two days, and he had slept in a valley throughout the freezing night as he hadn't the strength to reach the nearest village.

He rested with us before he could muster up the strength to tell us what had happened at Mantsonyane. The men had refused to take the building materials unless paid ten bob per donkey (standard price of material transport for traders is one-half that), and Molefi had finally, in exasperation, told them that he thought it would be OK. This news infuriates me.

Late this morning, the men from Mantsonyane showed up with the loaded donkeys, and I called the leader into the dispensary hut for a talk. I gave him a lecture on the self-help concept of our hospital, and made sure he understood that I knew the prices of transport in this country and wouldn't be snowed. I told him that we'd be damned if we would pay more than the normal prices for transport, and that we shouldn't even have to pay that; the hospital is for him, not for us.

He answered that he would transport the rest of the stuff at the standard rate of five bob per donkey if I would just pay him the ten bob per donkey for this load. I told him to go to hell. He therefore decided that he would take this load back to Mantsonyane; I told him that he may do what he damn well pleases, depending on whether or not he wants a hospital in his village. The people of Likhoiting will gladly take the materials if he doesn't want them.

After nearly two hours of trying to convince him why he should help himself and the other people of Sehlabeng, he agreed to transport all the stuff for five bob including this load he had just carried. Once I was sure he understood, I gave him ten bob per donkey in payment for this load, explaining that this was only because Molefi had made a promise and it wasn't my position to break it for him; but for the next trip, he gets nothing, zero, not a single cent.

We parted 'in peace', and I think he finally did get the gist of my words. It's nearly impossible though to get understanding even with any amount of careful explanation; it seems to be beyond the comprehension of these people that anyone should come here for any reason but to exploit them. Maybe I'm wrong, and this guy in fact does not understand—thinks that we are rich and must be out to become richer through the sweat of his people. It's hard to be sure.

This morning, Moromong, upon whom we can always depend for understanding and support, left for Mantsonyane with his own four donkeys. He doesn't want money for his labours.

I spoke with two local men, both of whom I know quite well as friends, about building. They are willing to build at a sub-economic wage, and will dig stones for us if we will only do them a favour, like getting them each a pair of overalls when the work is completed. It was one of the few encouragements we've had since returning here to start work. The problem now is that we are having difficulty locating a pick for digging stones. Such equipment isn't readily available in the mountains.

For all the discouragement, things are beginning to creep along here; Moromong should arrive with more building parts tomorrow.

A couple of days ago we managed to get two shovels and a crowbar from our friend Majara, so stone digging has begun. It is murderous work digging and breaking stones, but the two men who offered their help have been doing that all day each day without the aid of a pick, working steadily despite freezing weather and intermittent rain and ice storms. The evening we got the tools, they began arguing with us over money, and I finally told them, 'If you're interested in working, work; if you're not interested, go home—but don't stand here irritating us to death and wasting your own valuable time.' They walked off, and it was somewhat of a relief to find them working from sunrise the next morning, cutting stones at a remarkable pace.

Our friend Chief returned from a trip yesterday, all smiles at being back with us. He thinks that the *pitso* we plan will be a success, and that we won't have any difficulty getting help; he will back us if there is any problem. We had a great time talking with him, and joked as much as ever.

Last night Moromong arrived at about eleven with his four donkey-loads of building materials. I don't know what we would do without the help of people like him and Chief.

The weather has been bitterly cold what with winter approaching; the dampness is the worst of the cold. Icy rain has been falling each day, and the wetness permeates everything—clothes and blankets. This morning we awoke to see snow on all the mountain tops, just a thin layer but enough to make travel nearly impossible. It's beautiful to see the powdering of snow on the mountain peaks, fluffy clouds of mist drifting around them, but it isn't a happy omen of what we're in for soon.

The life here isn't bad for us, even with the freezing weather. One isn't constantly running into so much racial antagonism as in the lowlands, and the people here are generally kind and amazingly joyful, seemingly more joyful than ever in the contrast between their attitudes and the winter desolation. And the mountains themselves are always beautiful, though brutal. Mini, Chief, Mr. van Jaarsveld, Molefi and I get along well and have a good time every evening, our spirits heightened by short-wave music from Radio Tanganyika, Rhodesia and Mozambique. We struggle to hear the sounds of music through harsh static, and appreciate whatever we're lucky enough to make out.

During the days the clinic swarms with anxious patients. Here at Sehlabeng many people ride for hours to get medicines for sick people at their homes. We tell them time and again that we cannot dispense medicines without first seeing the patient, but they never understand. They insist first that the 'nurse' at the mission never refuses them; we explain that that doesn't make it correct to give out drugs without first seeing the patient—that the wrong medicine can kill a person, as can indiscriminately prescribed placebos such as the 'medicated wine' given out at high cost by the mission. They then tell us that the illness is simple enough: it is obviously 'bad bile' or 'blood behind the eyes'.

We have spread word that we are leaving on Wednesday unless something happens at the *pitso* scheduled for today. People are worried. They must be worried enough to do something constructive, however, if they want a hospital. The news that we might leave has had some rather embarrassing results.

Yesterday we received as presents from various local people piles of potatoes and two cabbages. Then in the afternoon came four kids of the local school-teacher with arms laden with gifts wrapped in paper. We opened the presents and found an amazing feast of gifts: a pile of tomatoes (we hadn't known they existed in the mountains), the ribs of a freshly slaughtered goat just loaded with fat, a pile of already cleaned potatoes, two cabbages of the largest possible size, and a thermos full of fresh milk still warm from the cow. Mini had recently treated the children, and this is a gift from their wealthy and generous father. We wrote him a note of thanks for the children to take back, but are embarrassed at the extent of the gift—and at his evident worry over our leaving, which most probably lies behind it.

A few days ago, Mini pointed to a man on a horse riding at a frantic pace through the veld, and said proudly that he is a man she has been treating for a serious heart condition. Yesterday the same man came to the tent to say hello, and I recognized him: last time Carl was here a patient was carried to him on a makeshift stretcher; the patient had had a heart attack and was in his last gasp. Carl did the best he could for him, and we found him accommodation at the chief's home, but there seemed little hope of his surviving. Now, as death, too, failed to stop him, we can't persuade him to slow down.

The two men working at the site have dug a tremendous pile of stones, despite all the freezing rain. This morning Moromong brought a pick which he had located at a distant village, and now things will move a bit faster. It's still slow going, however, without mass help.

The cold has been nearly unbearable—but people say that winter has hardly started. We've been spending a good deal of our time huddled over a dung fire with the rest of the villagers, nearly smothered by smoke, and in the evenings we close up the tent and let it fill with the steam of our breathing and cooking. The snow is melted today and the sun is strong, so it's not too bad, but yesterday the wind was shockingly icy from blowing over the snow. At night it is nearly impossible to get to sleep because of the shivery damp which penetrates even one's skin. We eat hot fat with dinner for warmth, and even the resulting heartburn is welcome for its heat.

Hardly anyone came to our *pitso*. By late afternoon we had about twenty villagers, including Chief Ntabe who is Chief Lepolisa's useless representative, and someone carrying a note from Chief Lepisa (a big important chief, oddly enough a woman—the one who eats people); Chief Lepisa said in her note that she would send her representative the next day. Our village headman Morena Pita was there, of course, but no other chiefs.

Chief Ntabe, a cruel-looking man, told me that he was in a hurry, so I began to discuss things with him, everyone crowded around, and this discussion became in itself the *pitso*.

The first thing Ntabe said to me was that we will probably finish the hospital and then claim that it belongs to us and not to the people as we have promised. When I asked him what grounds he had to make such an accusation, he said that he knows well enough not to trust outsiders; he pointed to the mission and said that the priest had said the same things we are now saying, and now the people cannot even use his mill. I told the chief bluntly that if he were going to sit here and talk to me as if I were a generality instead of an individual, he might as well scram. I am not his mission priest, but someone else with his own ideas and principles. He said, 'Well, we want a doctor here, so I won't argue with you.' I blew up, then spoke calmly, then exploded again—but I couldn't penetrate his prejudices.

We talked with the others present, and they all complained that the chiefs never tell them what is going on—saying they hadn't known what we were asking of them and that the people hadn't been informed properly of the *pitso*. I don't believe it, but am sure the fact is that they simply don't want to work for what they think they can have for nothing; as much as I tried to get them to the point of the matter—that if they want a hospital they can have it now by just working—they talked only about the chiefs' never telling them what's going on. Of all the people there, I found only one man willing to help; he is bringing his oxen on Saturday to drag stones to the site.

Finally I broke up the gathering as a waste when I got too sick of hearing 'look what the priest did', and so forth. All the time they were saying how much they want the hospital, but they don't do a damn thing about it—and with the exceptions of our personal friends here, they won't trust us enough. They cannot comprehend the idea of our being here actually to help them help themselves. And they don't understand that we haven't funds to give to them, nor with which to hire help.

This morning Chief Seliba, a representative of Chief Lepisa, came to see us. He's a nasty-looking man, and has a reputation to match—very proud of his position, very bossy. I played along with his pride, for we need someone who can give orders which will be obeyed; perhaps it is he.

We explained to him our difficulties, and he listened without apparent reaction. As we spoke, along came the man reputed to be the finest builder in this area of the mountains. Then and there, before Seliba, we bargained with him for his services, and he rejected all our offers. I turned back to the chief and said, 'See what I mean, Morena? Here's an excellent builder, he's badly needed for this work, but he isn't willing to work for our moderate wage. What can we do? We don't have any more to offer. How can we get this hospital built?'

With Chief Seliba's persuasion, the builder soon agreed to take our contract and start work as soon as there are enough stones.

Later, when Molefi and I walked past the rock quarry, we saw the two men we had hired working away feverishly next to a pile of already-cut rocks. They looked proud of their work.

This afternoon we were visited by Chief Tsoelike, Chief Tatolo, and the District Councillor Tara Tatolo—the first we've seen of them since the doctor tried unsuccessfully to land at Ha Tsoelika and we had to explain to them that the hospital must be at Ha Lepolesa. Now the three of them came riding up, an incongruous trio: Chief Tsoelike, the old man with his wire spectacles, who always sits quietly by during discussions, like a mummy; Chief Tatolo, fat and round, with the face and personality of a pouting, spoiled child; and intelligent, friendly, reasonable and rather dull

Tara Tatolo. We greeted each other warmly, having a genuine if vague liking for one another, and they came into the tent.

Tara Tatolo immediately asked me, 'Where is the hospital to be?' as if the situation must have changed by their will; they had been punishing us for the decision to build at Ha Lepolisa by staying away, figuring they'd force us to decide finally on Ha Tsoelike. I was surprised, and explained again that the doctor couldn't land at Ha Tsoelike, and therefore we had no choice but to decide on Ha Lepolisa. It's not a decision of whim, nor is it one which can be altered.

Chief Tatolo slapped his thigh, and looked away unhappily, stubbornly, a pout creasing his face. We tried to reason with him, but he wouldn't look at us, even when Tara Tatolo, his brother, tried to make him accept the situation. All our efforts were useless; he was throwing a tantrum—which could have serious consequences, for as area chief we need his support.

When we had used up all alternative approaches, I said to Chief Tatolo, 'Listen, you know we need your support to rally the people; we can't do without it. You stand by this hospital. Or forget about it—we'll leave.' He didn't react. Desperately I got up courage and said, 'You're acting like a spoiled child.' Tara Tatolo froze; even the lethargic Chief Tsoelike stiffened. I held my breath—and, by God, Chief Tatolo looked at me furiously, and then began to roar with laughter. I thought he was going to choke he laughed so hard, bent over in an agony of amusement. His spasms continued while Tara, Tsoelike and I recovered from our surprise, and then we were all hysterical, roaring with laughter, slapping each other on the back, nearly rolling on the ground it all seemed so terribly funny.

Molefi walked into the tent and found us at it; he stood there in utter confusion, until we saw him there and pulled ourselves together, slightly embarrassed and wondering at ourselves. Breathing hard, Chief Tatolo turned to me and said, 'What problems are you having getting the hospital built?' Relieved, I explained the difficulties of getting help of any kind, especially transporting of building materials. Chief Tatolo said strongly, 'I don't think you would have any trouble getting transport to Ha Tsoelike.' All of us laughed, more sanely now, and it was immediately agreed that Chiefs Tatolo and Tsoelike would send twenty donkeys of their own to Mantsonyane the day after tomorrow for the building materials, to be brought here, to Ha Lepolisa. Also, they will find men willing to work at the wage we have established. Finally the work is under way.

Chief had dinner with us again tonight; for a few nights we have eaten without him because he has had to work late in the fields. I told him how happy we are that he is again with us in the evenings, that we get lonely without him. He beamed. Later, when we had finished dinner and were listening on our radio to some Rock and Roll, Mini's weakness, Chief said to me, 'You mustn't listen to such music. It will remind you of your friends at home, and then we will lose you.' I was very touched, and knew he was right, it's nearly time for me to go home.

Yesterday, despite Carl's scheduled arrival, we had no hopes of seeing him, for storms were building in the distance, making the air turbulent, causing impossible flying conditions. The higher mountains around us were surrounded by dense clouds and mist. We gave up hope, and Mini went to the cliff at the beginning of the airstrip (our bathroom) while I began peeling potatoes for breakfast.

Then, amazingly, came the sound of a plane, and Carl came ripping over the mountains from the north, dodging piles of mist as he came. He invaded Mini's privacy as he came in to land (when she came to the tent later he greeted her with, 'I saw you,' and she covered her face in her embarrassment, giggling). I met the plane at the end of the strip; it was covered with mud as if it had been flying through a river. Carl opened the door, gave a sigh of relief, and greeted me warmly as if he had never really expected to arrive here alive.

Carl tells us that at other clinics things are going well too, that all over the country the people are building clinics and levelling airstrips, and then sending representatives to the lowlands to see him. At Mohokare, before a site was chosen for building, the people were coming out in force every day and piling up stones at all the possible building sites so that they would be ready to start work immediately when a site should finally be chosen. The village was cluttered with stones, ready to be moved as soon as Carl came to point his finger at a definite site. He's been seeing hundreds of enthusiastic patients at each clinic.

At Masianokeng things are bad, Carl had to report. The old spirit is gone. He has been fighting the committee every step of the way, and has no say in the development of the work. It's all he can do to make them realize the mountain people exist, much less to persuade some of the committee members that the mountain clinics require their intensified attention. He keeps asking himself how this work can possibly be directed by those who care so little about the patients that they've never even visited a mountain clinic. Carl is feeling discouraged by the direction BASOMED is taking, and asked me to return to the lowlands with him.

We arrived back at Masianokeng in the evening, just as preparations were in progress for a combination BASOMED meeting and cocktail party—the new face of socio-medical work apparently. Some things were the same: Rosalia's welcome, the excited youngsters, being with Carl again; but the house itself seemed different, despite Jan and Jackie's kindness—open arms in fact—and we were now somehow trespassers. Roslia watched our faces, and her reactions—shaking her head mournfully, casting sympathetic glances at us—reminded us that the work and Carl's home were no longer really his. We moved about in the house like ghosts.

The meeting in the centre room was more a social affair than a serious and productive evaluation of the work, but when a speech was made about the necessity to charge fees to patients for the sake of the organization, I could no longer hold back my protest, and I was asked to leave.

I was shocked, angered and I suppose somewhat humiliated as well. I quickly left the room, and Carl followed—not in protest, but to talk with me, seeing how upset I was.

I waited in his room. He came in and motioned me to sit, then poured two tots of brandy for us. I said, 'Carl, you see what BASOMED is becoming.' He didn't answer, but watched me seriously, with a trace of amusement too in his crazy, thoughtful way. I continued, 'They'll make it into a money-grinding business—the whole thing. One or two of the members of the committee are even against you, and would prostitute the most basic principles of your work—it's making me sick.' I rattled on, really angry, 'I'm not working for BASOMED. You know that very well—I'm working for you and the people in the mountains. Why do you let them get away with this?'

So many times I've argued with Carl about the necessity for him to assert his character without hesitation, told him that he has to quit worrying about whether he's being an egotist and just go ahead and rule over this work without doubting his right to hold a position of complete power. But he shakes his head and talks about humility, and lets others who haven't one-tenth his strength run over him. Now they're ruining his work, he's let them take over and still tries to believe that they're sincere and want to do the right thing. He told me now, 'Jeff, I often feel like dissolving the whole bloody business and carrying on alone, with you and a few other friends. The only help we need is that of the mountain people I often think. But we've established all these BASOMED clinics, and the people in the mountains are depending on us; we have to try to keep the work alive by continuing under these new conditions. For the first time these committee members are taking a part in the work; maybe now that they're involved, if we continue doing our old work in the mountains, they'll come to their senses and see the real importance of what we're doing.'

I shook my head, and he added, 'One of the things which has kept me going is a definite belief that goodness will conquer; the sincerity and depth of motivation behind our work should themselves stand as our work's best defence; this should keep it alive.' He cautioned me against being bitter, and pointed out optimistically that our mountain work is still going on strongly and effectively.

I admire him, I think his ideas are beautiful and his humility real and even noble—but I think he's destroying the value of his work by refusing to say, 'I'm right, I know I'm right, and I'll run this work the way I know it should be run.' But I believe in him—or am allowed to believe in him—more than he allows himself to believe in himself.

On Saturday morning, Carl and I again sat down to talk. We don't have the privacy we used to enjoy, but now managed to find a few minutes alone. I hesitantly told him, 'There's something I must talk to you about, a decision I've had to make.' He looked at me, knowing just what I was about to say, and I said it anyway. 'I think it's time for me to return to New York.' He said, 'I'll have to know the reasons why.' I told him that mostly I feel that my effectiveness here is very limited now, that there are personal reasons I have to return home and this seems the right time to do so. He said, 'My God, Jeff—you know you're the only person I can depend on, the only person I can turn to for understanding and support. I can't depend on anyone else.'

After a few minutes he said, 'We need time to talk. We should take a Sunday and fly somewhere in the mountains where we can just sit all day peacefully talking, discussing this and so many other things . . . that is, unless you've definitely made up your mind already.' I muttered, 'Well, I've pretty much made up my mind, but, you know, it depends a lot on what you feel is necessary.'

He laughed, saying, 'Well, there's a contradiction for you,' somewhat breaking the tension. I said, 'Well, it isn't an easy thing . . ' and he broke in, 'Yes, I know—our feelings are hard to express.'

Just a short while later, Carl announced that he was going to Bloemfontein, booked in by phone at a hotel there, and flew off. The next day when he returned, the first thing he said to me before we were interrupted by others was, 'I had a good time in the evening. I saw a movie you would have loved, about Ghandi. But I kept on wishing I had taken you along with me, and was depressed that I hadn't.' He's really lost, he has no home, even his work is no longer his own. He said nothing more about my leaving, and I went ahead and began making plans. In staying I make his distress over the future of the mountain work even worse by letting myself get even more upset than he. In leaving, no matter how or when, I let him down.

Carl arrived back from the mountains Saturday evening, after a six-day round of the clinics. He was in a state of collapse. Not surprising. This is his routine: on the first morning, after we pour boiling water over the plane wings to melt the layers of ice, he flies to the first clinic; he sees patients until dark, sometimes into the night, without resting; too tired to go through a dinner where he must eat while surrounded by staring multitudes, he collapses into bed (it's too cold to do anything else); with luck, he gets himself to sleep by ten or eleven in the night; he wakes up at four in the morning because of the penetrating cold; since it's much too cold to get up and make coffee or wash before sunrise (the water in the tent is solid ice anyhow), he lies in bed and soon finds himself brooding unhealthily; he gets up at sunrise, and is immediately surrounded by people, curious or in need of his help as a doctor and adviser; he sees a few emergency patients, then goes to the plane and warms it up for half an hour once it finally starts; and then he flies to the next clinic where he lives the identical routine over again. He certainly cannot maintain such a schedule, but it's more than I can do to convince him that he must stop before he kills himself. He tries to slow down, but faced with the people's need for a doctor, and troubled by organization problems, he drives himself into the mountain work relentlessly.

The committees at the clinics are working effectively and enthusiastically, running their own services; materials are being transported in mass to Sehlabeng already.

I wrote the BASOMED brochure, and to my surprise Jan liked it to the extent of getting tremendously excited over it. Last night I showed it to Carl, and he thought it effective—except that he thinks there is too much 'Dr. van Aswegen' in it. I answered, 'Dr. van Aswegen and the people he serves, what else is there? Let OXFAM write an organization brochure.' Carl looked at the brochure once more, and then to my surprise burst into one of his rare emotional crises, almost sobbing, 'Why, Jeff? Why must we present people overseas with a glamorous personality, or racial sensationalism, or the dangerous excitement of this work in order to get them to help and feel for other people?'

Carl went off to the mountains yesterday morning. The two weeks previous to that he had been completely closed in by snow, and had sat frustrated, thinking every day, 'There are a hundred people waiting at Sehlabeng, or a hundred waiting at Mohokare, and here I sit.' It would be no problem if we had radio units at all the clinics, as we had hoped we might before the Chamber of Mines recently rejected our application for a grant. Without radios, mountain work is frustrating and hazardous as can be.

Last Saturday, despite the snowy weather, Carl decided to go and do an especially important clinic at Machache. It seemed impossible to convince him not to, but after an hour or more of my insisting, to a point where I feared he might get angry, he said OK, he wouldn't go.

On Sunday afternoon I took advantage of a chance to get a lift to the Republic to say goodbye to Carl's parents, and to try to persuade them to understand that Carl is too busy to visit them often. Carl was relieved at my going, but warned me that I could expect to find his father angry at his long absence from home.

I reached his father on the phone from Maseru to tell him I was coming, and received irritable grunts in reply. When I arrived, at about eight in the evening, Mrs. van Aswegen threw her arms around me, but Mr. van Aswegen shook my hand coldly and said, bitterly, 'You visit us, but our son won't.' I explained to him what he knows very well, that Carl is terribly busy and, besides, doesn't yet have a visa for passing the new Basutoland border control established recently by the Republic, but he wouldn't listen. He said, 'If Carl were here working on his farm, as he should be doing, he wouldn't need a visa for anything.'

It was good to see them, and we sat up talking until one in the morning, but in many ways it was difficult. Mrs. van Aswegen probed me persistently for news of her son, which I gave her in bright terms, and Mr. van Aswegen cynically kept saying, 'Oh—Carl, Carl, Carl is all I hear' and made other somewhat brutal remarks. When I finally asked him directly, 'But aren't you proud of your son's work?' he answered, 'Proud? Why in hell should I be proud of Carl? He doesn't work. If he worked he'd have something to show for it. No MAN I know works for nothing.'

After we had gone off to bed, when I was just falling asleep, Mrs. van Aswegen timidly knocked at the door and asked me to please come out for a moment. I got dressed and followed her to the study, where sat Mr. van Aswegen; I was shocked to see his true expression, a face not hard and bitter, but softened and deep with feeling. Tears filled his eyes, and spilled down his leathery face as he said, 'We want you to have this money to thank you for all you've done for Carl.' He shoved a cheque for £20 into my hands. I just stood there, embarrassed by his having opened himself to me so suddenly, not wanting to take his money, so touched by his thought that I couldn't speak. He said, 'Don't take it as something material—it's from our hearts. We're just old farm people—we don't know any other way to express the thanks we feel in our hearts.' His tears abruptly disappeared, and he made one of his hard jokes; his face became a tough mask. Putting his arm over my shoulders, he said, 'You're so damn soft from that easy life you and Carl lead—you'll never be up in time for the train tomorrow morning. Get to bed.'

At five the next morning, Mr. van Aswegen woke me and we went in the freezing darkness to the station; as we drove he said, 'Thanks for coming all this way to see us and say goodbye. We're old people, and no one wants to see us. Not even our son.' I objected to his last phrase, for I now knew better than to accept it, and he cut me off with his laughter, and we understood each other. He put me on the train, and again with tears wetting his face, said, 'Thanks again. Carl needed you so badly, and will miss you so very much—he told me so himself. I hope we can see you again before we die . . .'

When I came into the house at Masianokeng, still confused and warmed by my moving experience with Carl's parents, tired and upset after a day's trip through the Republic, Jan and Jacki informed me that they are holding a big party for me on Saturday night with lots of people, and that it will be a great thing for BASOMED. I suppressed my rude desire to tell them to go to hell with their party, and gently as possible explained that while I am grateful for their thoughtfulness, I don't want a party, would find it most embarrassing. Jan told me teasingly that I have no say in the matter, but I wasn't kidding, and I told him so. I was adamant in both my appreciation and in my absolute refusal to go through with their plan, and we finally compromised that close friends only would be invited for drinks and dinner. Though misguided, it's a nice gesture on their part; they should know very well, however, than the last thing I want is a show of thanks.

This morning Carl had to go to Sehlabeng and Mafisa clinics and suggested that I come along to help him out. He knew that I wanted to say goodbye to my friends at Sehlabeng and to the mountains whose beauty I would also soon desperately miss. Since it was a perfectly clear and windless day over Masianokeng, we took off with some feeling of security.

Nearing the mountains at eight thousand feet, however, we flew into sudden turbulence so violent that it was nearly impossible to cross the escarpment where at ten thousand feet a wind of approximately fifty miles per hour nearly wrecked the aeroplane. We managed to get to Sehlabeng where we dropped a message explaining why we couldn't land—knowing the while that the people there are so reliant on the doctor's coming that they blame him and not the weather, despite all. Then we headed for Mafisa, but ran into such devastating turbulence that the doctor almost made an emergency landing on the mountain terrain; because there were two of us in the plane, he decided to attempt fighting his way back to Masianokeng rather than crash land. The return flight, which normally takes less than forty-five minutes, took us over ninety minutes because we had to battle with a furious head-wind, and at one point the plane nearly flipped on to its back. We climbed to twelve thousand feet, without oxygen, where the conditions were almost normal, thank goodness; an age later we landed safely at Masianokeng.

Saturday, the day of the goodbye party, was the roughest one. Jan and Jacki had invited about twenty of my closer friends; when they began arriving I was up to my neck retyping the corrected version of the brochure on to stencils. I had to stop my work to join the party at about four o'clock, and went off to put on some decent-looking clothes. Soon more cars started pulling up, numerous people coming despite a blizzard blowing outside. By five-thirty there were forty people, and we looked worriedly at our liquor supply; Jacki asked us to not eat too much at dinner, for she had prepared food for only an expected half this number of guests.

It was very warming, if embarrassing, that all my friends had turned up. Carl joined us, gave me a secret look of sympathy, and then began enjoying himself.

It was Cardwell, my closest friend, who started the speeches—despite my pleading with him not to. I cringed in a corner behind Julius Malie's back while Cardwell let loose, and thank goodness he was kind enough to keep it short. But he had started it, and everyone began standing up to say a few words. I was so terrified by the situation, and disgusted at the public praise, that I really couldn't appreciate the kindness of their words as I perhaps should have. It worked out well enough though when Mr. Khekhetla, the Minister of Health, put a bit of humour into the speeches by saying, 'I remember vividly one day when I was at a meeting with Jeff, sitting in the Resident Commissioner's office where Jeff was explaining a serious problem BASOMED was facing. I shall never forget Jeff's spiritedness, sincerity, and . . . uh . . . individuality. Well, perhaps I'd better not say any more about that.'

Carl was forced to speak, to his horror, but he finally got up, looked at me apologetically, and said, 'I find it very unfortunate that I must be put in a position of having to say goodbye to Jeff, especially formally and in public; it is no less than your asking me to say a speech of farewell to my brother. I will therefore reserve for now my deepest feelings, and will say here only that I refuse to acknowledge Jeff's leaving because I know that his spirit will remain as long as the spirit of our work, which he played such a large part in building materially and in principle, remains alive.'

Now the crowd called on me for a speech, and in my flushed state I simply told them that I have but one thing to express to them now, and that is my deep thanks for whatever support they have given our work and for their kindness to me.

For me the highlight of the evening was a long drunken conversation I had with Mr. Takele, our senior dispenser. He's a bright, straightforward guy, always ready to stand up for his ideas and prepared to boss even Carl around when angry. We are devoted to him, not only because of these admirable traits of character, but because they are combined with a most colourful oddity: the ability to be a thief with sincere feelings of justification. Takele will steal anything whenever he can. This evening, while in conversation with me, he would put his hand on my arm in drunken cameraderie, a moment later his hand would slip almost imperceptibly over the back of my hand, and before I knew it he would have taken my glass of brandy from me, downing it easily. This he did three times, each time with such naturalness that I watched with awe and cursing admiration.

Last night Carl and I spent the evening together over a bottle of gin—for which we had to search Basutoland, for it was a Sunday. We spoke mostly of the usual things, gently pushing off talk of my leaving, but once in a while he would say something like, 'I'm going to miss you so much,' or 'There's no one left to depend on.' At one point he told me, 'You mustn't be surprised if suddenly you receive a cable from me to say that I'm coming to New York to see you.' We didn't say very much, for words were inadequate, but we felt even closer than we ever have—as if our minds were working as one.

This morning Carl took a few pictures of me and had Jan take some of us together. After a while, fearing that I would miss my train, I started to get impatient and he pointedly ignored my agitation. Finally, when I was beginning to get upset, he said very calmly, his eyebrows raised, 'Really, Jeff, you're not going to get angry now, are you?' and we both laughed. Carl half-jokingly took from me the hat I had worn throughout the winter and gave me a small ashtray from his room, telling me that it must go wherever I go. Then he said, 'Strange that it is now we will truly get to know each other most intimately. I have so much to say to you which I am capable of saying only in writing—but, then perhaps we have managed to somehow say it to each other silently.'

With those words, we went out to the car where Jan was waiting, and just as it should have been—for we understood each other's feelings—Carl and I shook hands and said nothing but, 'Thanks'. I still can't comprehend that I won't see him for an indefinite time. We've shared what few people share in feeling, care and effort; we will somehow continue to do so, perhaps more strongly than ever.

I said goodbye to Rosalia, who cried and kept saying over and over again, 'When are you coming back—oh, Jeff, you've been so good, you've been so good, when are you coming back?' I felt helpless, and will miss her terribly too, but am comforted by knowing that she will soon convince herself that this is only another of my trips to the mountains. I hope she's right.

Epilogue I

On August 1st, 1963, I sat beside Dr. Albert Schweitzer in his room at Lambarene, Gabon. I was there as a personally invited guest on my way home, entrusted with the privilege of expressing Carl's feelings. I spoke with Dr. Schweitzer of Carl's Basutoland work and as if Dr. van Aswegen's very actions were thanks enough for all his inspiration and material support, Dr. Schweitzer adamantly refused to hear words of gratitude for all his help.

A week later, as I stepped into the boat which would take me away from the Schweitzer Hospital, I looked back and saw Dr. Schweitzer beam, wave goodbye again, and bustle off with steps confident and full of life—but rickety with age. In that moment I thought, with a shock, 'How very old he is!' I had known well his age to be eighty-eight, had seen the years reflected in his face, and had felt the wisdom of his words, but now for the first time I saw that the bend in his back and the quiver of exhaustion in his step were old—the steps of an old and tired man, not some sort of god. I looked once more at the sprawling hospital he had created of flimsy wood, rusty iron, and care for all humanity and life itself. He had cleared his way through the almost inconquerable jungle to establish his medical service for humanity, and in the same way he had cleared his way through the defensiveness and cynicism of humanity to establish a living philosophy of love.

Certainly he must be tired—for he's very human, and that's the beauty of his work. May everyone embarking on such work be able to make such claim.

Epilogue II

Since the writing of this book Dr. van Aswegen has resigned from BASOMED, leaving it administratively rich but run by a committee not one of whose members has the doctor's intimate knowledge of the mountains or the mountain people.

He refused to criticize publicly BASOMED, but instead moved to the lowland town of Leribe in hopes of somehow starting a small private practice from nothing. There he received immediate and overwhelming support from the local people. It was, in fact, the financial support from Basuto friends that enabled the doctor to make a new and successful beginning.

Today, in now independent Lesotho, formerly Basutoland, the doctor is working once again to bring health and self-respect within reach of the lowland and mountain people, struggling above the wreckage of his past years' labours to create anew their brilliance. He is succeeding.